Springer Japan KK

T. Akamizu, M. Kasuga
T.F. Davies (Eds.)

The Genetics of
Complex Thyroid Diseases

With 32 Figures, Including 1 in Color

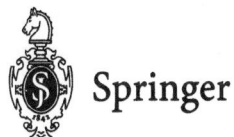 Springer

Takashi Akamizu, M.D.
Department of Medicine and Clinical Science, Kyoto University Graduate School of Medicine
54 Shogoin Kawahara-cho, Sakyo-ku, Kyoto 606-8507, Japan

Masato Kasuga, M.D.
Department of Internal Medicine, Kobe University School of Medicine
7-5-1 Kusunokicho, Chuo-ku, Kobe 650-0017, Japan

Terry F. Davies, M.D.
Division of Endocrinology and Metabolism
Mount Sinai School of Medicine
New York, NY 10029, USA

ISBN 978-4-431-68002-4   ISBN 978-4-431-67885-4 (eBook)
DOI 10.1007/978-4-431-67885-4

Typesetting: Camera-ready by the editors and authors

SPIN: 10854710

Preface

The rapid developments in molecular genetics have clarified many of the mutations in monogenic thyroid diseases over the last two decades; now the target of molecular thyroid genetics has become the oligogenic thyroid diseases. These include the autoimmune thyroid diseases and familial thyroid cancers, both of which are much commoner than the monogenic diseases. However, the methodological approach to the genetics of these more complex diseases is still far from being well established. Although the discovery of susceptibility genes has been partially accomplished in complex diseases such as asthma, Crohn's disease, and types I and II diabetes mellitus, the elucidation of susceptibility genes in complex diseases remains a major challenge.

This volume contains papers presented at the International Symposium on the Genetics of Complex Thyroid Diseases. This meeting was held in association with the International Thyroid Congress in Kyoto in October 2000 and supported in part by the Japan Intractable Diseases Research Foundation and Knoll Pharmaceuticals Inc. The symposium was the first international symposium concerning the genetics of complex thyroid diseases and was restricted to the study of the autoimmune thyroid diseases and familial thyroid cancer. Twenty distinguished researchers from the United States, the United Kingdom, France, Germany, Italy, and Japan were invited. Each presentation precipitated intense discussion and there was much consensus during the meeting. Nevertheless, this volume will leave the reader with a clear understanding of how little we still know.

On behalf of the organizing and executive committees, we wish to express our gratitude to those who participated in the conference and contributed to the preparation of these proceedings. Especially, we appreciated the assistance of Miss Maki Kouchi, who was very supportive in assembling the manuscripts. We believe this edited volume provides a comprehensive survey for those interested in the field of thyroid genetics.

The Editors

Organization of Symposium

ACTING PRESIDENT OF THE JAPAN INTRACTABLE DISEASES RESEARCH

Fumimaro Takaku Jichi Medical School, Tochigi, Japan

CHAIRMAN

Masato Kasuga Department of Internal Medicine, Kobe University School of Medicine, Kobe, Japan

Terry F. Davies Division of Endocrinology and Metabolism Mount Sinai School of Medicine, New York USA

ORGANIZING COMMITTEE

Terry F. Davies Division of Endocrinology and Metabolism Mount Sinai School of Medicine, New York, USA

Takashi Akamizu Department of Medicine and Clinical Science Kyoto University Graduate School of Medicine, Kyoto, Japan

Yaron Tome Division of Endocrinology, Diabetes and Bone Diseases, Department of Medicine, Mount Sinai School of Medicine, New York, USA

Stephen Gough Department of Medicine, University of Birmingham, Birmingham, UK

Klaus Badenhoop Department of Endocrinology, Centre Internal Medicine (ZIM), Frankfurt am Main, Germany

James A. Fagin Division of Endocrinology and Metabolism University of Cincinnati, Ohio, USA

EXECUTIVE COMMITTEE

Masato Kasuga	Department of Internal Medicine, Kobe University School of Medicine, Kobe, Japan
Takashi Akamizu	Department of Medicine and Clinical Science Kyoto University Graduate School of Medicine, Kyoto, Japan
Nobuyuki Amino	Laboratory Medicine, Osaka University Graduate School of Medicine, Osaka, Japan
Junji Konishi	Department of Nuclear Medicine, Kyoto University Graduate School of Medicine Kyoto, Japan
Toru Mori	Kyoto Senbai Hospital, Kyoto, Japan
Shigenobu Nagataki	ITC, AOTA, Hiroshima, Japan
Hisao Seo	Division of Endocrinology and Metabolism Research Institute of Environmental Medicine Nagoya University, Nagoya, Japan
Fumimaro Takaku	Jichi Medical School, Tochigi, Japan
Terry F. Davies	Division of Endocrinology and Metabolism Mount Sinai School of Medicine, New York USA

SECRETARIAT

Takashi Akamizu	Department of Medicine and Clinical Science Kyoto University Graduate School of Medicine, Kyoto, Japan

Acknowledgments

The editors gratefully acknowledge the support of the following organizations and individuals

HOST ORGANIZATIONS

The Japan Intractable Diseases Research Foundation
The Japanese Ministry of Health and Welfare
Knoll Pharmaceuticals Inc.

SECRETARY-GENERAL

Shukue Azuma

Contents

Part 2 Familial Thyroid Cancers

Contributors

Part 1

Autoimmune Thyroid Diseases

GENETIC DISSECTION OF FAMILIAL AUTOIMMUNE THYROID DISEASES USING WHOLE GENOME SCREENING

Yaron Tomer MD, FACP
Division of Endocrinology, Diabetes and Bone Diseases, Department of Medicine, Mount Sinai School of Medicine, New York, New York.
Correspondence to: Dr. Y. Tomer,
Division of Endocrinology and Metabolism, Box 1055, Mount Sinai Medical Center, One Gustave L. Levy Place, New York, N.Y. 10029, USA
TEL: (212) 241-7085 **FAX:** (212) 241-4218
E-mail: Yaron.Tomer@mssm.edu

Key words

Graves' disease, autoimmune thyroid disease, Hashimoto's thyroiditis, anti-thyroid autoantibodies, CTLA-4, microsatellite marker, linkage study, HLA

INTRODUCTION

The autoimmune thyroid diseases (AITDs) including Graves' disease (GD) and Hashimoto's thyroiditis (HT) are some of the commonest human autoimmune diseases and are responsible for significant morbidity in pre-menopausal women [1;2]. The AITDs, are caused by immune responses to the thyroid gland. In Graves' disease the autoimmune process results in the production of thyroid stimulating antibodies and leads to hyperthyroidism, while in Hashimoto's thyroiditis the end result is thyroid cell death and hypothyroidism [reviewed in [3] and [4]]. While the clinical presentations of GD and HT are different, they share many features in common: (1) Humoral and cellular immune reaction to thyroid antigens [5]; (2) Infiltration of the thyroid by T cells which are biased in their V gene use [6]; (3) Female preponderance of

3

the diseases [7]; and (4) Strong familial predisposition (reviewed in [8]). However, the cause of the immune response to thyroid antigens in AITD remains unknown. Research into the pathogenesis of AITD has focused on the possible precipitating environmental insults (such as infection [9]) and on understanding the genetic predisposition to the disease. The recent advances in our understanding of the genetic susceptibility to AITD is the focus of this review.

EVIDENCE FOR A GENETIC SUSCEPTIBILITY TO AITD

Abundant epidemiological data point to a strong genetic contribution to the development of AITD. These epidemiologic data are derived from studies of unrelated individuals, family studies and twin studies.

Secular trends in the incidence of AITD: Studies from different geographic regions have shown a relatively similar incidence and prevalence of GD in different populations [2;7;10;11]. The comparable prevalence and incidence in geographically different populations suggested a significant genetic effect on the development of the disease because these populations were exposed to different environmental factors. Moreover, the incidence has not changed in the past several decades [12], again pointing to a strong genetic influence on disease development. The incidence rates of diseases with strong environmental influences are expected to change over time while the incidence rates of diseases with strong genetic influences should not change as much.

Familial clustering of GD: The familial occurrence of GD has been recognized by investigators for many years. More than 50 years ago it was recognized that a familial predisposition can be found in approximately 60% of cases with Graves' disease [13]. Martin [14] found that 20 of 90 (22%) of patients with Graves' disease had relatives with Graves' disease. Moreover, several thyroid abnormalities have been reported in relatives of patients with Graves' disease [15],[16],[17]; most commonly the presence of thyroid autoantibodies which were reported in up to 50% of the siblings of patients with AITD [18],[16],[19]. Hall and Stanbury [20] found clinical thyroid disease in 33% of siblings of patients with Graves' or Hashimoto's diseases. Additionally, they found 56% of siblings to be thyroid antibody positive and in almost all cases the parents of an affected individual were also positive [20]. While the sibling risk of developing autoimmune thyroid disease [8] has not been calculated directly, it was estimated to be >15 for Graves' disease from

4

published data [21]. Even though this is only a rough estimate, it is notable that the value is relatively high suggesting a strong genetic contribution to the development of Graves' disease.

Twin studies: Twin studies can provide information concerning the inheritance of a disease and may yield certain quantitative evaluations on the role of heredity in relation to exogenous factors. The twin method is based upon comparison of the concordance (simultaneous occurrence) of a given disease among monozygotic (MZ) twins and among dizygotic (DZ) twins. It must be emphasized that MZ twins are not identical in their immune repertoire due to somatic recombinations which T and B cells undergo throughout life as well as individual immune experiences which influence the immune repertoire. Therefore, part of the observed discordance between MZ twins may also be due to the discordance in their immune repertoire. In the largest twin study of Graves' disease, performed in Denmark, the concordance rate for MZ twins was 35%, and for DZ twins it was 3% [22]. For Hashimoto's thyroiditis the concordance rates were 38% for MZ twins and 0 for DZ twins [23], and for TAb's the concordance rates were 80% for MZ twins and 40% for DZ twins [23]. Thus, the twin data have indicated that, despite differences in their immune repertoire, there remains a substantial inherited susceptibility to AITD, presumably related to both immune and non-immune genes.

Thyroid autoantibodies: Autoantibodies to thyroglobulin (Tg) and thyroid peroxidase (TPO) have been widely used to show the population at most risk for the development of autoimmune thyroid disease (AITD). Anti-thyroid autoantibodies (anti-thyrogloblin and anti-thyroid peroxidase) have been found in up to 50% of the siblings of patients with AITD [16;18;19;24], in contrast to a prevalence of 7-20% in the general population [10]. These findings have also been found in different populations such as the Japanese [25] and British [20]. In one study, it was found that thyroid autoantibodies were almost always present in one of the parents of an affected individual with AITD [20]. These data suggested an inherited influence on the production of anti-thyroid antibodies compatible with dominant inheritance [26]. Indeed, segregation analyses in a panel of families with thyroid antibodies also suggested a Mendelian dominant pattern of inheritance for the tendency to develop anti-thyroid antibodies [27].

5

METHODS FOR IDENTIFYING THE AITD GENES

Several approaches are being taken to identify the susceptibility genes for AITD. The two most popular approaches are candidate gene analysis and whole genome screening.

Analysis of candidate genes: Candidate genes are genes of known sequence and location which could, theoretically be involved in disease pathogenesis. If a candidate gene is the cause of the disease, then markers close to that gene should segregate with the disease within a family. Since the basic abnormality in AITD is an immune response against thyroid cells, candidate genes for GD include genes that control antibody responses (e.g. the immunoglobulin gene complex and genes responsible for B cell growth factors), genes that control T cell responses (e.g. the HLA region, the T-cell receptor genes and genes responsible for T cell growth factors), and genes encoding the target autoantigens (thyroglobulin [Tg], thyroid peroxidase [TPO], TSH receptor [TSHR]). Several of these genes have now been studied for their possible role in the genetic susceptibility to AITD.

Whole genome screens: Linkage studies can also be used for genome-wide genetic screening. The technique of whole genome screening involves typing of individuals in large families with AITD for polymorphic markers. These markers are then analyzed for linkage with AITD in the tested families. If linkage to one or more markers is established it can be concluded that a susceptibility gene for the disease is located near that marker. The markers chosen may span the whole human genome at distances that will enable detection of linkage to susceptibility genes located between any two of them. The polymorphic markers most often used in genome-wide scans are the microsatellites, which are regions in the genome composed of short repetitive units (e.g. CA-repeats). Microsatellites are abundant and uniformly distributed throughout the genome at distances of less than 1 million base pairs [28]. A set of 400 microsatellite markers is now commercially available and they span the whole human genome at distances short enough (< 10 centimorgan) to detect linkage to any locus between them. Once a suspected locus is located, it can be further narrowed using markers that are more closely spaced, and the gene region identified. In order to identify complex disease genes it has been necessary to use large numbers of families and to use strict conservative phenotype definitions.

WHOLE GENOME SCREENING IN AUTOIMMUNE THYROID DISEASES

The initial whole genome scan: We performed the first whole genome screening in AITD in a dataset of 56 multiplex families (354 individuals) [29;30] (**Table 1**). The whole genome screening revealed seven loci which showed evidence for linkage with AITD: three loci were linked to Graves' disease, GD-1 on chromosome 14, GD-2 on chromosome 20, and GD-3 on chromosome X; Two loci were linked to IIT: IIT-1 on chromosome 13, and HT-2 on chromosome 12. One locus (AITD-1) was linked with both Graves' and Hashimoto's diseases [29], and another locus (TAb-1) was linked with thyroid antibodies [31].

Other screenings: In order to confirm that a locus is indeed linked with AITD another independent linkage study should also demonstrate linkage at the same locus [32]. So far only GD-2 and TAb-1 have been replicated by other groups [33;60]. In addition, we are currently analyzing a second dataset of 46 multiplex families (186 individuals).

Conclusions from the genome scans in AITD: The genome scans performed in AITD families have shown that the genetic contribution to the development of GD involves several genes with varying effects. Our data also showed evidence for interactions between these genes. Some of the AITD susceptibility loci were common to both GD and HT (AITD-1, TAb-1) while others were unique to each diseases (e.g. GD-1, HT-1). This may imply that the development of GD and HT involves common genes for thyroid autoimmunity but that the specific phenotype requires participation of other disease specific genes. It is also likely that environmental factors may also play a role in determining the resultant phenotype in a genetically susceptible individual.

PUTATIVE AITD SUSCEPTIBILITY GENES

The major histocompatibility genes

Association of HLA with Graves' disease (Table 2):   Graves' disease was found to be associated with HLA-DR3 [34;35]. The frequency of DR3 in GD patients was 40-55% and in the general population 20-30% giving a relative risk for people with HLA-DR3 of 2.1-3.7 [35;36] (Table 2). The HLA associations were found to be different in other ethnic groups. In the Japanese population GD was associated with HLA-B35 [37], and in the Chinese population an increased frequency of HLA-Bw46 has been reported [38]. In African-Americans no overall susceptibility could be associated with any DR allele, although subdivision of the patients revealed that DRw6 was associated with thyroid antibody formation [39]. Among Caucasians, it has recently been shown that the DRB1*0301 allele was the primary susceptibility allele for GD, and other associated alleles were most likely due to linkage disequilibrium with DRB1*0301 [40].

Association of HLA with Hashimoto's thyroiditis: Data on HLA haplotypes in Hashimoto's thyroiditis are less definitive than in GD. A general methodological problem has been that while the diagnosis of GD is relatively straight forward, the definition of HT has been more controversial. This has reflected the fact that the disease encompasses a spectrum of manifestations, ranging from the simple presence of TAb's with focal lymphocytic infiltration, to the presence of goitrous or atrophic thyroiditis, characterized by gross thyroid failure. While initial studies failed to demonstrate HLA associations for any A- B- or C- antigens [41], an association with HLA DR5 was observed in goitrous HT [42] and with DR3 in atrophic HT [43]. More recently, an association has been reported between HT and HLA-DQw7 (DQB1*0301) [44;45]. Associations of HT with other HLA haplotypes have also been reported in different ethnic populations, e.g. HLA-DRw53 in Japanese, and HLA-DR9 in Chinese (for review see [46]).

HLA linkage studies in AITD: Studies in HT have not demonstrated evidence for linkage to HLA genes, again supporting the notion that the HLA genes are not of major importance in the pathogenesis of HT. Similarly, linkage studies in GD have been mostly negative except for one study in a relatively small group of selected sib-pairs (reviewed in [47]). Therefore, although certain HLA genes conferred an increased risk of developing GD and HT, they were of minor significance in the overall susceptibility to AITD.

Conclusions on HLA: The HLA genes have shown consistent associations with GD, but no linkage with GD or HT. Moreover, the risk of developing GD in HLA-identical siblings was only 7%, which was not significantly different from the general risk in siblings [48]. Furthermore, this was much lower than the 35% concordance for MZ twins described earlier. Therefore, we have to conclude that the HLA genes are not the primary GD genes, and are more likely to be modulating genes increasing the risk for AITD conferred by other genes.

Mechanisms of HLA influences: The mechanisms by which HLA associations confer disease susceptibility in GD are now beginning to be understood. In order for T cells to recognize and respond to an antigen there has to be recognition of a complex between the antigenic peptide and an HLA class II molecule [49]. It is thought that different HLA alleles have different affinities to autoantigens (e.g. thyroid antigens) which are recognized by T cell receptors [50]. Thus, certain alleles may permit the autoantigen to fit in the antigen binding groove inside the HLA molecule and to be recognized by the T-cell receptor while others may not [51]. Furthermore, such fits may be of variable ease. It has been postulated that if a certain HLA allele allowed only weak (low affinity) binding of an autoantigen to the HLA molecule then the autoantigen would not be presented to T cells in the thymus during embryonic life. The result would be that the T cell clone recognizing this autoantigen would not be deleted and would survive able to induce an autoimmune condition later in life. Conversely, HLA alleles that confer strong binding to a specific autoantigen will allow its presentation to T cells in the thymus and these autoreactive T cells would be deleted by apoptosis and would not be able to induce an autoimmune condition. Even if an autoreactive T-cell clone was not deleted it cannot react with thyroid antigens unless these antigens are presented to it in sufficient concentration. Thus, mechanism for autoantigen presentation must exist within the thyroid gland of GD patients. One potential intrathyroidal mechanism not utilizing professional antigen presenting cells (APC's) may be through aberrant expression of HLA class II molecules on thyrocytes [52].

The CTLA-4 gene

CTLA-4 association studies in AITD (Table 3): Recently, there have been several reports demonstrating a weak association between the CTLA-4 gene and the AITDs [53-56]. Earlier studies found an association between a microsatellite marker located near the CTLA-4 gene and GD, giving a relative risk of 2.1 to 2.8 [53;56]. With the identification of an alanine/threonine (G/A) polymorphism inside the CTLA-4 leader peptide, this polymorphism was also tested for association with the AITDs. The ala (G) polymorphism was found to be associated with GD with a relative risk of 2.0 [55] (Table3). These reports have been consistent in several populations [53;56]. Two groups have also recently claimed that the G allele of the CTLA-4 SNP was specifically associated with Graves' ophthalmopathy (GO) [57;58]. We recently tested the CTLA-4 A/G_{49} SNP in GO and found no specific association of the G allele with GO beyond the association with GD and AITD [59]. Thus the bulk of the data suggests that the G allele of the CTLA-4 SNP is associated with AITD in general and not with any specific AITD phenotype.

CTLA-4 linkage studies in AITD: Recently, Vaidya et al. [60] reported linkage in addition to association of the CTLA-4 region on chromosome 2q33 with GD. The linkage became stronger in families with AITD, rather than just GD, suggesting a more general role for CTLA-4 in thyroid autoimmunity and not a specific predisposition to GD. In keeping with these observations we found strong evidence that the CTLA-4 gene region was linked with the production of thyroid autoantibodies [31]. Further analysis showed a much higher frequency of the G allele of the CTLA-4 SNP in the linked families compared with the unlinked families and controls [31]. These results suggested that CTLA-4 actually conferred a general susceptibility to thyroid antibody production and that the development of clinical disease (Graves' or Hashimoto's diseases) required the participation of other disease-specific genes and environmental factors.

Mechanisms of CTLA-4 influences: APC's activate T cells by presenting to the T cell receptor an antigenic peptide bound to an HLA class II protein on the cell surface. However, a second signal is also required for T cell activation and these co-stimulatory signals may be provided by the APC's themselves or other local cells [61]. The co-stimulatory signals are provided by a variety of proteins (e.g. B7-1, B7-2, CD-40) which are expressed on APC's and interact with receptors (CD28, CTLA-4, and CD-40L) on the surface of CD4+ T-lymphocytes during antigen presentation [61]. Whereas, the binding of B7 to CD28 on T cells co-stimulates T cell activation, the binding of B7 to CTLA-4 is thought to down regulate T-cell activation and induce tolerance. The suppressive effects of CTLA-4 on T cell activation have raised the possibility that mutations altering CTLA-4 function could lead to the development of autoimmunity. Indeed, DeGroot and colleagues have shown that the G allele of the CTLA-4 A/G_{49} SNP reduced the suppressive effects of CTLA-4 on T-cell activation [62]. These results may support a general role for CTLA-4 in the development of autoimmunity.

CONCLUSIONS

The AITDs are multifactorial disease which are caused by genetic susceptibility and environmental triggers. Various epidemiological and genetic techniques can be employed to study the genetic contribution to disease development. Most epidemiologic data support an important genetic contribution to the development of AITD. The genetic susceptibility to AITD involves several genes with varying effects. Some AITD susceptibility genes are most likely immune modifying genes which increase the susceptibility to autoimmunity in general (e.g. HLA, CTLA-4) while others may be thyroid specific. These genes probably act in concert to increase the autoimmune reactions in susceptible individuals and direct them towards the thyroid.

Acknowledgements:

We thank Dr. David Greenberg for his teaching, support and ever ready help in our joint studies. We also thank Erlinda Concepcion for her exceptional technical support. Our studies were supported in part by: DK35764, DK45011 & DK52464 from NIDDK (to TFD), and DK02498 from NIDDK (to YT).

Table 1: Two point and multipoint LOD scores at the 6 loci which were found to be linked with AITD.

Locus	Marker Name	Chromo-some	2-Point LOD	Multipoint LOD	Penetrance/ Inheritance	NPL
AITD-1	D6S257	6p	2.2	2.9	0.3/Rec.	2.3
GD-1	D14S81	14q31	2.1	2.5	0.3/Rec.	1.9
GD-2	D20S195	20q11.2	3.2	3.5	0 .3/Rec.	2.4
GD-3	DXS8020	Xq21	1.9	2.5	0.4/Rec.	1.8
HT-1	D13S173	13q32	1.8	2.1	0.3/Rec.	1.0
HT-2	D12S351	12q22	1.7	2.3*	0.8/Rec.	0
TAb-1	D2S325	2q33	3.6	4.2*	0.8/Dom.	2.2

* Heterogeneity LOD score (i.e. only a subset of the families is linked)

Table 2: Some of the important HLA association studies in Graves' disease Performed in Caucasians.

Country	Ethnic Group	No. Of Patients	HLA Allele	RR	Reference
Canada	Caucasians	175	B8 DR3	3.1 5.7	[63]
England	Caucasians	127	B8 DR3	2.77 2.13	[64]
France	Caucasians	94	B8 DR3	3.4 4.21	[65]
Hungary	Caucasians	256	B8 DR3	3.48 4.80	[66]
Ireland	Caucasians	86	B8 DR3	2.5 2.6	[67]
Newfoundland	Caucasians	133	DR3	4.57	[68]
Sweden	Caucasians	78	B8 DR3	4.4 3.9	[69]
USA	Caucasians	65	DR3	3.38	[35]
England	Caucasians	120	DQA1 *0501	3.8	[70]
USA	Caucasians	94	DQA1 *0501	3.71	[71]

Table 3: Some of the important CTLA-4 association studies in Graves' disease.

Polymorphism/ Marker	Country	Ethnic Group	Dis.	No.	RR[*]/ P value	Ref
CTLA-4(AT)	USA	Caucasians	GD	133	2.82	[53]
CTLA-4(AT)	Hong-Kong	Chinese	GD	94	p=0.037	[54]
CTLA-4(AT)	UK	Caucasians	GD	112	2.1	[56]
CTLA-4(AT)	Japan	Japanese	GD	62	NS*	[72]
Thr/Ala $(A/G)_{49}$	Germany	Caucasians	GD	305	2.0	[55]
Thr/Ala $(A/G)_{49}$	Japan	Japanese	GD	153	2.64	[73]
Thr/Ala $(A/G)_{49}$	UK	Caucasians	GD	94	p=0.003	[57]
C-T (-318)	UK	Caucasians	GD	188	NS	[74]
	China	Chinese	GD	98	NS	

[*]RR-relative risk, NS-not significant

REFERENCES

1. Jacobson DL, Gange SJ, Rose NR, Graham NM (1997) Epidemiology and estimated population burden of selected autoimmune diseases in the United States. Clin Immunol Immunopathol 84:223-243.

2. Vanderpump MPJ, Tunbridge WMG, French JM, Appleton D, Bates D, Clark F, Grimley Evans J, Hasan DM, Rodgers H (1995) Tunbridge F, Young ET. The incidence of thyroid disorders in the community: a twenty-year collow-up of the Whickham survey. Clin Endocrinol (Oxf) 43:55-68.

3. Davies TF (1996) The pathogenesis of Graves' disease. In: Braverman LE, Utiger RD, editors. Werner and Ingbar's The Thyroid: a fundamental and clinical text. Philadelphia: Lippincott-Raven, 525-536.

4. Weetman AP (1996) Chronic autoimmune thyroiditis. In: Braverman LE, Utiger RD, editors. Werner and Ingbar's The thyroid. Philadelphia: Lippincott-Raven, 738-748.

5. Weetman AP, McGregor AM. (1984) Autoimmune thyroid disease: developments in our understanding. Endocr Rev 5:309-355.

6. Davies T, Concepcion E, Ben-Nun A, Graves P, Tarjan G. (1993) T-cell receptor V gene usage in autoimmune thyroid disease: Direct assessment by thyroid aspiration. Journal of Clinical Endocrinology and Metabolism 76:660-666.

7. Mogensen EF, Green A.(1980) The epidemiology of thyrotoxicosis in Denmark. Incidence and geographical variation in the Funen region 1972-1974. Acta Med Scand 208:183-186.

8. Tomer Y, Barbesino G, Greenberg DA, Davies TF (1997) The immunogenetics of autoimmune diabetes and autoimmune thyroid disease. Trends Endocrinol Metab 8:63-70.

9. Tomer Y, Davies TF (1993) Infection, Thyroid Disease and Autoimmunity. Endocrine Rev 14:107-120.

10. Tunbridge WMG, Evered DC, Hall R, Appleton D, Brewis M, Clark F, Evans JG, Young E, Bird T, Smith PA (1977) The spectrum of thyroid disease in a community: the Whickham survey. Clin Endocrinol Oxf 7:481-493.

11. Furszyfer J, Kurland LT, McConahey WM, Elveback LR (1970) Graves' disease in Olmsted County, Minnesota, 1935 through 1967. Mayo Clin Proc 45:636-644.

12. Furszyfer J, Kurland LT, McConahey WM, Woolner LB, Elveback LR (1972) Epidemiologic aspects of Hashimoto's thyroiditis and Graves' disease in Rochester, Minnesota (1935-1967), with special reference to temporal trends. Metabolism 21(3):197-204.

13. Bartels ED (1941) Twin Examinations: Heredity in Graves' disease. Copenhagen: Munksgaad, 32-36.

14. Martin L. (1945) The heredity and familial aspects of exophathalmic goitre and nodular goitre. Q J Med 14:207-219.

15. Tamai H, Ohsako N, Takeno K, Fukino O, Takahashi H, Kuma K, Kumagai LF, Nagataki S. (1980) Changes in thyroid function in euthyroid subjects with family history of Graves' disease; a followup study of 69 patients. J Clin Endocrinol Metab 51:1123-1128.

16. Chopra IJ, Solomon DH, Chopra U, Yodhihara E, Tersaki PL, Smith F (1977) Abnormalities in thyroid function in relatives of patients with Graves' disease and Hashimoto's thyroiditis: lack of correlation with inheritance of HLA-B8. J Clin Endocrinol Metab 45:45-54.

17. Tamai H, Kumagai LF, Nagataki S (1986) Immunogenetics of Graves' disease. In: McGregor AM, editor. Immunology of endocrine diseases. Lancaster, U.K.: MTP Press 123-141.

18. Volpe R (1985) Autoimmune thyroid disease. In: Volpe R, editor. Autoimmunity and endocrine disease. New York: Marcel Dekker, 109-285.

19. Burek CL, Hoffman WH, Rose NR. (1982) The presence of thyroid autoantibodies in children and adolescents with AITD and in their siblings and parents. Clin Immunol Immunopathol 25:395-404.

20. Hall R, Stanbury JB (1967) Familial studies of autoimmune thyroiditis. Clin Exp Immunol 2:719-725.

21. Vyse TJ, Todd JA (1996) Genetic analysis of autoimmune disease. Cell 85:311-318.

22. Brix TH, Kyvik KO, Christensen K, Hegedus L (2001) Evidence for a major role of heredity in Graves' disease: a population- based study of two Danish twin cohorts. J Clin Endocrinol Metab 86(2):930-934.

23. Brix TH, Kyvik KO, Hegedus L (2000) A population-based study of chronic autoimmune hypothyroidism in Danish twins. J Clin Endocrinol Metab 85(2):536-539.

24. Hall R, Dingle PR, Roberts DF (1972) Thyroid antibodies: a study of first degree relatives. Clin Genet 3:319-324.

25. Aho K, Gordin A, Sievers K, Takala J (1983) Thyroid autoimmunity in siblings: a population study. Acta Endocrinol Suppl. 251:11-15.

26. Jaume JC, Guo J, Pauls DL, Zakarija M, McKenzie JM, Egeland JA, Burek CL, Rose NR, Hoffman WH, Rapoport B, McLachlan SM (1999) Evidence for genetic transmission of thyroid peroxidase autoantibody epitopic "fingerprints". J Clin Endocrinol Metab 84(4):1424-1431.

27. Phillips DIW, Prentice L, McLachlan SM, Upadhyaya M, Lunt PW, Rees Smith B (1991) Autosomal dominant inheritance of the tendency to develop thyroid autoantibodies. Exp Clin Endocrinol 97:170-172.

28. Weber JL (1990) Human DNA polymorphisms based on length variations in simple- sequence tandem repeats. Genome Analysis 1:159-181.

29. Tomer Y, Barbesino G, Greenberg DA, Concepcion ES, Davies TF. (1999) Mapping the major susceptibility loci for familial Graves' and Hashimoto's diseases: Evidence for genetic heterogeneity and gene interactions. J Clin Endocrinol Metab 84:4656-4664.

30. Tomer Y, Barbesino G, Greenberg DA, Concepcion ES, Davies TF. (1998) A new Graves disease-susceptibility locus maps to chromosome 20q11.2. Am J Hum Genet 63:1749-1756.

31. Tomer Y, Greenberg DA, Barbesino G, Concepcion ES, Davies TF. (2001) CTLA-4 and not CD28 is a susceptibility gene for thyroid autoantibody production. J Clin Endocrinol Metab 86:1687-1693.

32. Lander E, Kruglyak L (1995) Genetic dissection of complex traits: guidelines for interpreting and reporting linkage results. Nature Genet 11:241-247.

33. Pearce SH, Vaidya B, Imrie H, Perros P, Kelly WF, Toft AD, (1999) McCarthy MI, Young ET, Kendall-Taylor P. Further evidence for a sus-

ceptibility locus on chromosome 20q13.11 in families with dominant transmission of Graves disease [letter]. Am J Hum Genet 65(5):1462-1465.

34. Farid NR, Sampson L, Noel EP, Barnard JM, Mandeville R, Larsen B, Marshall WH, Carter ND (1979) A study of human D locus related antigens in Graves' disease. J Clin Invest 63:108-113.

35. Mangklabruks A, Cox N, DeGroot LJ (1991) Genetic factors in autoimmune thyroid disease analyzed by restriction fragment length polymorphisms of candidate genes. J Clin Endocrinol Metab 73:236-244.

36. Volpe R (1990) Immunology of human thyroid disease. In: Volpe R, editor. Autoimmunity in endocrine disease. Boca Raton: CRC Press, 73.

37. Kawa A, Nakamura S, Nakazawa M, Sakaguch S, Kawabata T, Maeda Y, Kanehisa T (1997) HLA-BW35 and B5 in Japanese patients with Graves' disease. Acta Endocrinol (Copenh) 86:754-757.

38. Chan SH, Yeo PP, Lui KF, Wee GB, Woo KT, Lim P, Cheah JS. (1978) HLA and thyrotoxicosis (Graves' disease) in Chinese. Tissue Antigens 12:109-114.

39. Sridama V, Hara Y, Fauchet R, DeGroot LJ (1987) HLA immunogentic heterogenity in Black American pateitns with Graves' disease. Arch Intern Med 147:229-231.

40. Zamani M, Spaepen M, Bex M, Bouillon R, Cassiman JJ (2000) Primary role of the HLA class II DRB1*0301 allele in Graves disease. Am J Med Genet 95(5):432-437.

41. Irvine WJ, Gray RS, Morris PJ, Ting A (1978) HLA in primary atrophic hypothyroidism and Hashimoto goitre. J Clin Lab Immunol 3:193-195.

42. Farid NR, Sampson L, Moens H, Barnard JM (1981) The association of goitrous autoimmune thyroiditis with HLA-DR5. Tissue Antigens 17:265-268.

43. Moens H, Farid NR, Sampson L, Noel EP, Barnard JM (1978) Hashimoto's thyroiditis is associated with HLA-DRw3. N Engl J Med 299:133-134.

44. Wu Z, Stephens HAF, Sachs JA, Biro PA, Cutbush S, Magzoub MM, Becker C, Schwartz G, Botazzo GF (1994) Molecular analysis of HLA-

DQ and -DP genes in caucasoid patients with Hashimoto's thyroiditis. Tissue Antigens 43:116-119.

45. Badenhoop K, Schwartz G, Walfish PG, Drummond V, Usadel KH, Bottazzo GF (1990) Susceptibility to thyroid autoimmune disease: molecular analysis of HLA-D region genes identifies new markers for goitrous Hashimoto's thyroiditis. J Clin Endocrinol Metab 71:1131-1137.

46. Weetman AP (1991) Autoimmune Endocrine Disease. Cambridge: Cambridge University Press

47. Tomer Y, Davies TF (2000) The genetics of familial and non-familial hyperthyroid Graves' disease. In: Rapoport B, McLachlan SM, editors. Graves' disease: Pathogenesis and treatment. Boston: Kluwer Academic Publishers 19-41.

48. Stenszky V, Kozma L, Balazs C, Rochlitz S, Bear JC, Farid NR (1985) The genetics of Graves' disease: HLA and disease susceptibility. J Clin Endocrinol Metab 61:735-740.

49. Buus S, Sette A, Grey HM (1987) The interaction between protein-derived immunogenic peptides and Ia. Immunol Rev 98:115-141.

50. Nelson JL, Hansen JA (1990) Autoimmune disease and HLA. CRC Crit Rev Immunol 10:307-328.

51. Faas S, Trucco M (1994) The genes influencing the susceptibility to IDDM in humans. J Endocrinol Invest 17:477-495.

52. Davies TF (1985) Co-culture of human thyroid monolayer cells and autologous T cells: impact of HLA class II antigen expression. J Clin Endocrinol Metab 61:418-422.

53. Yanagawa T, Hidaka Y, Guimaraes V, Soliman M, DeGroot LJ. (1995) CTLA-4 gene polymorphism associated with Graves' disease in a caucasian population. J Clin Endocrinol Metab 80:41-45.

54. Nistico L, Buzzetti R, Pritchard LE, Van der Auwera B, Giovannini C, Bosi E, Larrad MT, Rios MS, Chow CC, Cockram CS, Jacobs K, Mijovic C, Bain SC, Barnett AH, Vandewalle CL, Schuit F, Gorus FK, Tosi R, Pozzilli P, Todd JA (1996) The CTLA-4 gene region of chromosome 2q33 is linked to, and associated with, type 1 diabetes. Hum Mol Genet 5:1075-1080.

55. Donner H, Rau H, Walfish PG, Braun J, Siegmund T, Finke R, Herwig J, Usadel KH, Badenhoop K (1997) CTLA4 alanine-17 confers genetic susceptibility to Graves' disease and to type 1 diabetes mellitus. J Clin Endocrinol Metab 82:143-146.

56. Kotsa K, Watson PF, Weetman AP (1997) A CTLA-4 gene polymorphism is associated with both Graves' disease and autoimmune hypothyroidism. Clin Endocrinol 46:551-554.

57. Vaidya B, Imrie H, Perros P, Dickinson J, McCarthy MI, Kendall-Taylor P, Pearce SH (1999) Cytotoxic T lymphocyte antigen-4 (CTLA-4) gene polymorphism confers susceptibility to thyroid associated orbitopathy [letter]. Lancet 354(9180):743-744.

58. Buzzetti R, Nistico L, Signore A, Cascino I (1999) CTLA-4 and HLA gene susceptibility to thyroid-associated orbitopathy [letter]. Lancet 354(9192):1824.

59. Villanueva RB, Inzerillo AM, Tomer Y, Barbesino G, Meltzer M, Concepcion ES, Greenberg DA, Maclaren N, Sun ZS, Zhang DM, Tucci S, Davies TF (2000) Limited genetic susceptibility to severe graves' ophthalmopathy: No role for ctla-4 and evidence for an environmental etiology. Thyroid 10:791-798.

60. Vaidya B, Imrie H, Perros P, Young ET, Kelly WF, Carr D, Large DM, Toft AD, McCarthy MI, Kendall-Taylor P, Pearce SH (1999) The cytotoxic T lymphocyte antigen-4 is a major Graves' disease locus. Hum Mol Genet 8(7):1195-1199.

61. Reiser H, Stadecker MJ (1996) Costimulatory B7 molecules in the pathogenesis of infectious and autoimmune diseases. N Engl J Med 335:1369-1377.

62. Kouki T, Sawai Y, Gardine CA, Fisfalen ME, Alegre ML, DeGroot LJ (2000) CTLA-4 Gene Polymorphism at Position 49 in Exon 1 Reduces the Inhibitory Function of CTLA-4 and Contributes to the Pathogenesis of Graves' Disease. J Immunol 165(11):6606-6611.

63. Farid NR, Stone E, Johnson G (1980) Graves' disease and HLA: clinical and epidemiologic associations. Clin Endocrinol (Oxf) 13:535-544.

64. Kendall-Taylor P, Stephenson A, Stratton A, Papiha SS, Perros P, Roberts DF (1988) Differentiation of autoimmune ophthalmopathy from

Graves' hyperthyroidism by analysis of genetic markers. Clin Endocrinol (Oxf) 28:601-610.

65. Allannic H, Fauchet R, Lorcy Y, Gueguen M, Le Guerrier AM, Genetet B (1983) A prospective study of the relationship between relapse of hyperthyroid Graves' disease after antithyroid drugs and HLA haplotype. J Clin Endocrinol Metab 57:719-722.

66. Stenszky V, Kozma L, Balazs C, Rochkitz S, Bear JC, Farid NR (1985) The genetics of Graves' disease: HLA and disease susceptibility. J Clin Endocrinol Metab 61:735-740.

67. McKenna R, Kearns M, Sugrue D, Drury MI, McCarthy CF (1982) HLA and hyperthyroidism in Ireland. Tissue Antigens 19:97-99.

68. Payami H, Joe S, Thomson G (1989) Autoimmune thyroid disease in Type 1 diabetes. Genetic Epidemiology 6:137-141.

69. Dahlberg PA, Holmlund G, Karlsson FA, Safwenberg J (1981) HLA-A, -B, -C and -DR antigens in patients with Graves' disease and their correlation with signs and clinical course. Acta Endocrinol (Copenh) 97:42-47.

70. Barlow ABT, Wheatcroft N, Watson P, Weetman AP (1996) Association of HLA-DQA1*0501 with Graves' disease in English caucasian men and women. Clin Endocrinol 44:73-77.

71. Yanagawa T, Mangklabruks A, Chang YB, Okamoto Y, Fisfalen M-E, Curran PG, DeGroot LJ (1993) Human histocompatibility leukocyte antigen-DQA1*0501 allele associated with genetic susceptibility to Graves' disease in a caucasian population. J Clin Endocrinol Metab 76:1569-1574.

72. Sale MM, Akamizu T, Howard TD, Yokota T, Nakao K, Mori T, Iwasaki H, Rich SS, Jennings-Gee JE, Yamada M, Bowden DW (1997) Association of autoimmune thyroid disease with a microsatellite marker for the thyrotropin receptor gene and CTLA-4 in a Japanese population. Proc Assoc Am Physicians 109:453-461.

73. Yanagawa T, Taniyama M, Enomoto S, Gomi K, Maruyama H, Ban Y, Saruta T (1997) CTLA4 gene polymorphism confers susceptibility to Graves' disease in Japanese. Thyroid 7:843-846.

74. Heward JM, Allahabadia A, Carr-Smith J, Daykin J, Cockram CS, Gordon CBAH, Franklyn JA, Gough SCL (1998) No evidence for allelic association of human CTLA-4 promoter polymorphism with autoimmune thyroid disease in either population-based case-control or family-based studies. Clin Endocrinol 49:331-334.

GENOME SCREENING FOR GRAVES' DISEASE SUSCEPTIBILITY LOCI IN U.K. FAMILIES

B. Vaidya, H. Imrie, P. Kendall-Taylor, S.H.S. Pearce
Department of Endocrinology, University of Newcastle, Newcastle upon Tyne, U.K
Correspondence: Dr. B. Vaidya
Department of Endocrinology, University of Newcastle, Newcastle upon Tyne, NE2 4HH, U.K.
Tel. (44) 191 222 8026   Fax. (44) 191 222 0723
Email. bvaidya@hgmp.mrc.ac.uk

Abstract

Defining the susceptibility loci for complex multigenic disorders, such as Graves' disease (GD), remains difficult. We have screened diverse chromosome regions of the human genome in 68 multiplex white GD families (75 GD affected sib-pairs) from the U.K. in an attempt to identify susceptibility loci for GD. This genome screening has, to date, shown evidence to support linkage of GD at four chromosome regions: 2q33 (CTLA-4), 18q21 (IDDM6), 6p21 (MHC), and Xp11 (IDDMX). There was weak evidence to suggest linkage to chromosome 20q13 (GD2), but only in a sub-set of 12 families with an apparent dominant pattern of inheritance. Our results show that (a) loci at different chromosome regions confer susceptibility to GD, (b) some of these GD loci coincide with the susceptibility loci for type 1 diabetes and other autoimmune disorders, (c) there is genetic heterogeneity between the U.K. and other populations with GD, and (d) the family ascertainment criteria may affect the ability to detect linkage to some susceptibility loci.

Key Words

Graves' disease, autoimmune thyroid diseases, CTLA-4, AITD, chromosome2q31-q36, thyroid-associated orbitopathy, TAO, chromosome 18q21 chromosome 6p21, X chromosome, chromosome 14q31, chromosome 20q13, IDDM6, IDDM12

Introduction

Graves' disease (GD) is an organ-specific autoimmune disorder, which is characterised by a diffuse goitre and thyroid hormone oversecretion due to the stimulation of the thyrotropin receptor (TSH-R) by thyroid-stimulating autoantibodies. It is a common disorder predominantly affecting females. A survey in the town of Whickham (north east of England) found that about 2% of women and 0.2% of men had biochemical evidence of thyrotoxicosis, the majority of which is caused by GD (Tunbridge et al., 1977). Although the exact aetiology of GD remains unclear, it is believed that GD is caused by a complex interaction between genetic, environmental and constitutional factors. In recent years, there has been a huge effort to define genetic factors conferring susceptibility to GD. Here, we review the findings of our genetic linkage studies in multiplex GD families from U.K.

FAMILIAL CLUSTERING OF GRAVES' DISEASE

Twin studies and familial risk studies have provided good evidence for the genetic basis of GD. Recent population-based twin studies from Denmark have shown a significantly higher proband-wise concordance rate of GD in monozygotic twins (35%) than in dizygotic twins (3%) (Brix et al., 2001). Likewise, several familial risk studies have shown clustering of GD in families (reviewed in Brix et al., 1998). It has been estimated that a female sib of a GD proband is 10-15 times more likely to develop this disease as compared to the general population (sib risk ratio, lambda-s, 10-15) (Vyse & Todd, 1996; Brix et al. 1998).

We have reassessed the degree of familial clustering of GD and other autoimmune disorders in our GD cohort. The prevalence of GD, autoimmune hypothyroidism (AH) and other autoimmune disorders were analysed in first-degree relatives of 190 unselected GD probands recruited sequentially from outpatient clinics of the Newcastle hospitals. Of these, 33 (17%) and 37 (19%) GD probands had first-degree relatives who were also affected with GD and AH, respectively (Table 1). Fifteen (7.9%) GD probands were found to have sibs concordant for GD. Thus, assuming the population prevalence of overt GD as 0.8% based on the Whickham survey (Tunbridge et al., 1977), the sib risk ratio (lambda-s) for GD in our population is about 10 (concordance risk in sibs/ population prevalence, 7.9/0.8) (Risch, 1987). It should, however, be noted that this is likely to be an underestimate, as the diagnosis of GD in some of the unaffected sibs may be unknown, while others may develop GD in the future. In addition to the autoimmune thyroid diseases (AITD), there was also an increased prevalence of other autoimmune disorders, particularly type 1 diabetes (T1DM) and rheumatoid arthritis (RA), in the relatives of GD probands (Table 2). This is consistent with previous observations (Torfs et al., 1986; Payami et al. 1989), which suggest that different autoimmune disorders could have a common genetic predisposition.

GENOME LINKAGE SCREENING FOR GRAVES' DISEASE SUSCEPTIBILITY LOCI

Although GD, like the majority of autoimmune disorders, is inherited as a complex multigenic trait (Vyse & Todd, 1996), the genetic loci conferring susceptibility to this disease remain largely undefined. Therefore, in an attempt to identify susceptibility loci for GD, we have screened diverse chromosome regions of the human genome in a homogeneous cohort derived from 68 multiplex white GD families from the U.K. (Pearce et al., 1999; Vaidya et al., 1999a, 2000; Imrie et al., 2001). These families were ascertained by the presence of at least two sibs affected with GD, and were recruited from the north east of England and the adjacent Lothian region of Scotland. Linkage analysis was performed primarily using non-parametric methods in up to 75 sib-pairs with GD and 83 sib-pairs with AITD (GD and AH) derived from these families. A non-parametric method assesses the proportion of alleles shared by affected sib-pairs at a locus. Under random Mendelian expectation, full sib-pairs are expected to share 0, 1 and 2 alleles identical by descent 25%, 50% and 25% of the time, respectively. A significant excess of allele sharing between sib-pairs as compared to this random expected allele sharing (25%, 50%, 25% distribution) indicates linkage. In contrast to the classical parametric method, a non-parametric method is 'model-free' and does not require specification of mode of inheritance and penetrance for analysis, which may be difficult in complex traits. Therefore, it is regarded as the preferred method for linkage analysis of complex disorders (Lander & Schork, 1994). We have used the GENEHUNTER version 2 (Kruglyak et at., 1996) and MAPMAKER/SIBS (Kruglyak & Lander, 1995) programmes to compute linkage analysis. The results of our linkage analyses at different chromosome regions are summarised below.

The cytotoxic T lymphocyte antigen-4 (CTLA-4) region of chromosome 2

The chromosome 2q31-q36 region contains several candidate susceptibility loci for GD and other autoimmune disorders. Among these, one strong candidate locus is the cytotoxic T lymphocyte antigen-4 (CTLA-4) gene (2q33), which encodes a key negative regulator of T cell activation (Waterhouse et al., 1995). Alleles of the CTLA-4 gene have been shown to be linked to and associated with T1DM, and this locus has been designated IDDM12 (Nisticò et al., 1996; Marron et al., 2000). Two further putative T1DM loci, IDDM7 (2q31) and IDDM13 (2q35) have also been mapped to this region (Copeman et al., 1995; Morahan et al., 1996). Furthermore, both case-control and intra-familial association studies have consistently demonstrated an association of alleles of the CTLA-4 gene with GD in different populations (Yanagawa et al., 1995, 1997; Donner et al., 1997; Kotsa et al., 1997; Heward et al., 1999; Akamizu et al., 2000). However, the previous linkage studies have failed to confirm CTLA-4 as a susceptibility locus for GD (Tomer et al., 1997; Barbesino et al., 1998).

We have analysed our GD families for linkage to thirteen polymorphic markers across a 50 cM region of chromosome 2q31-q36, which encompassed the IDDM7, CTLA-4 (IDDM12) and IDDM13 loci (Figure 1). Non-parametric linkage analysis, designating only GD subjects as affected, showed evidence of linkage with a peak multipoint non-parametric linkage score (NPL) of 3.07 (p=0.001) at the marker D2S117, which is within 2.5 cM of CTLA-4 (Figure 1) (Vaidya et al., 1999a). Designation of all AITD subjects (GD and AH) as affected increased the peak NPL to 3.43 (p=0.0004) (Figure 1), suggesting homogeneity between GD and AH at this locus. We have estimated that the CTLA-4 locus (lambda-s 2.2) may confer up to one-third of the total genetic susceptibility to GD in our population. In addition to the CTLA-4 locus, linkage analysis of GD sib-pairs also showed a separate but smaller peak (NPL 1.54, p=0.06) at the IDDM13 region, suggesting that there may be an independent susceptibility locus in this region (Figure 1).

In order to fine-map the linkage in the region, we performed an intrafamilial association study of the chromosome 2q31-q36 markers by using unaffected sibs as controls (Curtis, 1997). This showed an association of GD with the G allele of the exon 1 CTLA-4A/G polymorphism (p=0.005), and the 112 mobility unit (mu) allele of the microsatellite CTLA-4(AT)n polymorphism (p=0.02) (Table 3), suggesting that a susceptibility polymorphism(s) lies at, or close to, the CTLA-4 gene. In addition, the frequency of the 149 mu allele of D2S137 at chromosome 2q35 (IDDM13) was also found to be higher in GD probands than in their unaffected sibs (p=0.014) (Table 3).

In case-control studies, we found that CTLA-4 alleles also confer susceptibility to the presence and severity of thyroid-associated orbitopathy (TAO) in patients with GD (Vaidya et al., 1999b). This CTLA-4 allelic association with TAO was independent of other risk factors for TAO, including male sex, advancing age, smoking status and previous radioiodine treatment. A subsequent study from Italy also supported the allelic association of CTLA-4 with TAO (Buzzetti et al., 1999), although another study from U.S.A. could not find this association (Villanueva et al., 2000). Recently, Heward et al. (1999) have demonstrated that GD patients with the GG genotype of the CTLA-4A/G polymorphism have more severe biochemical hyperthyroidism at presentation. Together, these observations suggest that different CTLA-4 alleles, by modulating immune responses differentially, may influence both the development and severity of GD phenotypes, including the development of extrathyroidal manifestations, such as TAO.

The chromosome 18q21 (IDDM6) region

In view of the familial clustering of GD with other autoimmune disorders, we have screened our GD families for linkage to different putative loci that have been found linked to T1DM and other autoimmune disorders (Table 4). Two-point linkage analysis by using single markers showed NPL of less than 1.0 at all these loci, except at IDDM6 (NPL 1.57) and AITD1 (NPL 1.23). We further examined the IDDM6 region by genotyping 11 microsatellite markers spanning 48 cM across chromosome 18q12-q22 (Vaidya et al., 2000). Multipoint linkage analysis, designating all AITD sib-pairs as affected, showed evidence of linkage with a peak NPL of 3.46 (p=0.0003) at the marker D18S487 (Figure 2). Designation of only GD cases as affected showed a peak NPL of 3.09 (p=0.001). Furthermore, both intrafamilial and case-control association analyses have shown an association of the 119 mu allele of D18S487 with GD, which is the same allele that has been found to be associated with T1DM (Merriman et al., 1997). It is estimated that this locus (lambda-s 1.8) confers about one-quarter of the total genetic susceptibility to GD in our population. Apart from T1DM and GD, recent genome-wide scans in rheumatoid arthritis (Cornelis et al., 1998), systemic lupus erythematosus (Shai et al., 1999) and Crohn's disease (Duerr et al., 2000) have also shown some evidence of linkage to this chromosome locus. Taken together, these observations suggest that this chromosome region may harbour an important autoimmunity locus.

The major histocompatibility complex (MHC) region of chromosome 6

The major histocompatibility complex (MHC), also known as the human leukocyte antigen (HLA) region in humans, is located on chromosome 6p21. Many studies in white populations have now confirmed the association of GD with the HLA-DR3 carrying haplotypes (reviewed in Brix et al., 1998). In contrast, three parametric linkage studies from the same laboratory have been unable to confirm linkage of GD to MHC, however these studies were small (Roman et al., 1992; O'Connor et al., 1993) or used mixed AITD families with cases of both GD and AH being classified as affected (Tomer et al., 1997). Recently, by using the transmission disequilibrium test in a cohort of GD families, Heward et al. (1998) have shown evidence of linkage of MHC to GD.

We have analysed the chromosome 6p21 region spanning the MHC locus by genotyping five microsatellite markers (Vaidya et al., 1999a). This showed some evidence to support linkage of GD to MHC, with a peak multipoint NPL of 1.95 (p=0.026) occurring at the markers D6S273 and TNFA. It is estimated that the MHC region confers about 18% of total genetic susceptibility to GD in our population. Thus, it appears that the contribution of MHC in the genetic susceptibility to GD is modest as compared to T1DM, where MHC has been demonstrated as the most important locus, contributing more than one-third of the total genetic susceptibility (Davies et al., 1994).

Chromosomes 14q31 (GD1), 20q13 (GD2) and Xq21 (GD3)

A recent genome-wide scan on multiplex AITD families suggested the presence of three GD susceptibility loci: on chromosome 14q31 about 25 cM away from TSH-R (designated GD1), on chromosome 20q13 (GD2) and on chromosome Xq21 (GD3) (Tomer et al., 1999). We have examined these putative loci in our GD families in an attempt to confirm linkage. A 36 cM region of chromosome 14q31-q33 encompassing the TSH-R gene and the GD1 locus was analysed by genotyping 8 polymorphic markers (Imrie et al., 2001). This showed no evidence of linkage of GD to this region in our cohort (peak NPL 0.36, p=0.36). In addition, we were unable confirm the previously reported association of GD with the T allele of the TSH-R P52T polymorphism (Cuddihy et al., 1995).

We examined an 83 cM region of the X chromosome encompassing GD3 on Xq22 and a putative T1DM locus (IDDMX) (Cucca et al., 1998) on Xp11 by genotyping 12 polymorphic markers (Figure 3) (Imrie et al., 2001). There was no evidence to support linkage of GD to the GD3 region. However, we found a peak multipoint NPL of 2.21 (p=0.014) at marker DXS8083 (more than 35 cM away from GD3), suggesting the existence of a GD susceptibility locus near IDDMX. The peak NPL increased to 3.18 (p=0.001) in data that have been conditioned for allele sharing at the CTLA-4 locus, which suggests a possible epistatic (multiplicative) interaction between these loci.

We genotyped five microsatellite markers in the chromosome 20q13 region to examine linkage at the GD2 locus (Pearce et al., 1999). There was no evidence to support linkage at this locus (peak NPL 0.1). In fact, we were able to exclude a hypothetical GD locus with a lamba-s >2.5 from this chromosome region. As our family ascertainment strategy (at least two affected sibs with GD) was different from that used by Tomer et al. (1999) (at least two affected first-degree relatives with AITD), it was speculated that their cohort is likely to contain many more affected parent-offspring kindreds, enriching for dominant susceptibility alleles. To test this hypothesis, we analysed linkage in a subgroup of 12 families with apparent dominant transmission (parent to offspring) of GD, which showed modest evidence suggestive of linkage with a peak NPL of 2.02 (p=0.023). However, as the number of families in this analysis is very small, this result should be interpreted cautiously. Similar analyses of apparent dominant GD families for the GD1 and GD3 loci did not show evidence of linkage.

LINKAGE STUDIES OF GRAVES' DISEASE IN A GLOBAL CONTEXT

Our genome linkage screening and other recent familial linkage reports have, thus far, provided varying degrees of evidence for several putative GD susceptibility loci in different populations, thus confirming the multigenic inheritance of GD (Table 5). Many of these putative GD susceptibility loci overlap with loci found to be linked to other autoimmune disorders, in particular T1DM (Table 5). This may explain the majority of the concordance of different autoimmune disorders in the same patients or their families. The evidence for some of these loci has been observed in two independent datasets, for example, MHC (Heward et al., 1998; Vaidya et al., 1999a), CTLA-4 (Heward et al., 1999, Vaidya et al., 1999a), and possibly GD2 (Tomer et al., 1998b; Pearce et al., 1999). Linkage of other loci, namely GD1 (Tomer et al., 1997, 1998a), GD3 (Barbesino et al., 1998), 18q21 (Vaidya et al., 2000) and Xp11 (Imrie et al., 2001) has been found in one dataset and these await confirmation in other populations. Furthermore, the evidence for some loci was found in one population, but not in the other population studied. For example, the linkage of GD to MHC and CTLA-4 was clearly observed in the families from U.K. (Heward et al., 1998, 1999; Vaidya et al., 1999a), but this was not detected by the studies from the U.S.A. group (Tomer et al., 1997, 1999; Barbesino et al., 1998). However, the U.S.A. group has recently reported linkage of the CTLA-4 locus with thyroid antibody production (Tomer et al., 2001). Similarly, the linkage of GD to the GD1 and GD3 loci shown by the studies from the U.S.A. group (Tomer et al., 1997, 1998a, 1999; Barbesino et al., 1998) was not confirmed by our studies (Imrie et al., 2001) (Table 5).

There are several possible reasons for the apparently conflicting findings of the studies from different centres. Firstly, replication of a linkage result for a complex disorder usually requires a much larger data-set than the initial study (Suarez & Hampe, 1994), and therefore the studies from different centres lacked the power to reproduce all of each-other's linkage results. Secondly, different phenotype selection (for example, GD or AH) may critically affect the ability to detect linkage at some loci. The families in the studies from U.S.A. are phenotypically more heterogeneous, with a large number of subjects with AH, and are derived from a geographically diverse background. This phenotypic heterogeneity could have affected the power of their studies to detect linkage at certain loci, such as MHC (Roman et al., 1992; Tomer et al., 1997), which shows allelic heterogeneity between GD and AH (GD is associated with HLA-DR3, while AH shows association with HLA-DR4/DR5). Thirdly, the ascertainment strategies in the recruitment of families may have a significant effect on the ability to detect a given susceptibility locus for complex disorders, as we encountered in the analysis of GD2. Fourthly, the studies from U.S.A. have mainly used parametric methods for linkage analysis, which may be sensitive to misspecification of background allele frequencies, penetrances and the mode of inheritance (Lander & Schork, 1994). Finally, there may be genuine genetic heterogeneity between our U.K. GD population and other populations with GD.

Summary and Future Directions

Identification of a "pathogenic" disease susceptibility allele for a complex genetic disease using reverse genetic approaches remains an elusive goal, although there is some progress in other fields (Horikawa et al., 2000). The linkage of GD to the CTLA-4 and IDDM6 regions is likely to stand the test of time, and a susceptibility allele or haplotype with an influence on many auto-immune disorders is likely to be identified from each of these regions in the future. The other regions of genetic linkage identified for GD need further fine-mapping studies with larger datasets of GD subjects, to confirm linkage and identify intervals of allelic association. However, knowledge about the genetics of autoimmune thyroid diseases has progressed considerably in the last six years, and clinically relevant advances are likely to accrue from the eventual identification of the common GD susceptibility alleles.

Acknowledgements

We are grateful to Drs P Perros, WF Kelly, D Carr, ET Young, DM Large, AD Toft and J Dickinson for allowing us to study their patients. This work was supported by the Wellcome Trust.

References

1. Akamizu T, Sale MM, Rich SS, et al (2000) Association of auto-immune thyroid disease with microsatellite markers for the thyrotropin receptor gene and CTLA-4 in Japanese patients. Thyroid 10:851-8.
2. Barbesino G, TomerY, Concepcion ES, et al (1998) Linkage analysis of candidate genes in autoimmune thyroid disease. II. Selected gender-related genes and the X chromosome. J Clin Endocrinol Metab 83:3290-5.
3. Becker, KG (1999) Comparative genetics of type 1 diabetes and autoimmune disease: common loci, common pathways? Diabetes 48:1353-8.
4. Brix TH, Kyvik KO, Hegedus L (1998) What is the evidence of genetic factors in the etiology of Graves' disease? A brief review. Thyroid 8:727-34.
5. Brix TH, Kyvik KO, Christensen K, et al (2001) Evidence for a major role of heredity in Graves' disease: a population-based study of two Danish twin cohorts. J Clin Endocrinol Metab 86:930-4.

6. Buzzetti R, Nisticò L, Signore A, et al (1999) CTLA-4 and HLA gene susceptibility to thyroid-associated orbitopathy. Lancet 354:1824.

7. Copeman JB, Cucca F, Hearne CM, et al (1995) Linkage disequilibrium mapping of a type 1 diabetes susceptibility gene (IDDM 7) to chromosome 2q31-q33. Nature Genet 9:80-5.

8. Cornelis F, Faure S, Martinez M, et al (1998) New susceptibility locus for rheumatoid arthritis suggested by a genome-wide linkage study. Proc Natl Acad Sci U S A 95:10746-50.

9. Cucca F, Goy JV, Kawaguchi Y, et al (1998) A male-female bias in type 1 diabetes and linkage to chromosome Xp in MHC HLA-DR3-positive patients. Nat Genet 19:301-2.

10. Cuddihy RM, Dutton CM, Bahn RS (1995) A polymorphism in the extracellular domain of the thyrotropin receptor is highly associated with autoimmune thyroid disease in females. Thyroid 5:89-95.

11. Curtis D (1997) Use of siblings as controls in case-control association studies. Ann Hum Genet 61:319-33.

12. Davies JL, Kawaguchi Y, Bennett ST, et al (1994) A genome-wide search for human type 1 diabetes susceptibility genes. Nature 371:130-6.

13. Donner H, Rau H, Walfish PG, et al (1997) CTLA4 Alanine-17 confers genetic susceptibility to Graves' disease and to type 1 diabetes mellitus. J Clin Endocrinol Metab 82:143-6.

14. Duerr RH, Barmada MM, Zhang L, et al (2000) High-Density Genome Scan in Crohn Disease Shows Confirmed Linkage to Chromosome 14q11-12. Am J Hum Genet 66:1857-62.

15. Heward JM, Allahabadia A, Daykin J, et al (1998) Linkage disequilibrium between the human leukocyte antigen class II region of the major histocompatibility complex and Graves' disease: replication using a population case control and family-based study. J Clin Endocrinol Metab 83:3394-7.

16. Heward JM, Allahabadia A, Armitage M, et al (1999) The development of Graves' disease and the CTLA-4 gene on chromosome 2q33. J Clin Endocrinol Metab 84:2398-401.

17. Horikawa Y, Oda N, Cox NJ, et al (2000) Genetic variation in the gene encoding calpain-10 is associated with type 2 diabetes mellitus. Nat Genet 26:163-75.

18. Imrie H, Vaidya B, Perros P, et al (2001) Evidence for a Graves' disease susceptibility locus at chromosome Xp11 in a U.K. population. J Clin Endocrinol Metab 86:626-30.

19. Jacobson DL, Gange SJ, Rose NR, et al (1997) Epidemiology and estimated population burden of selected autoimmune diseases in the United States. Clin Immunol Immunopathol 84:223-43.

20. Kotsa K, Watson PF, Weetman AP (1997) A CTLA-4 gene polymorphism is associated with both Graves disease and autoimmune hypothyroidism. Clin Endocrinol 46:551-4.

21. Kruglyak L, Lander ES (1995) Complete multipoint sib-pair analysis of qualitative and quantitative traits. Am J Hum Genet 57:439-54.

22. Kruglyak L, Daly MJ, Reeve-Daly MP et al (1996) Parametric and nonparametric linkage analysis: A unified multipoint approach. Am J Hum Genet 58:1347-63.

23. Lander ES, Schork NJ (1994) Genetic dissection of complex traits. Science 265:2037-48.

24. Marron MP, Zeidler A, Raffel LJ, et al (2000) Genetic and physical mapping of a type 1 diabetes susceptibility gene (IDDM12) to a 100-kb phagemid artificial chromosome clone containing D2S72-CTLA4-D2S105 on chromosome 2q33. Diabetes 49:492-9.

25. Merriman T, Twells R, Merriman M, et al (1997) Evidence by allelic association-dependent methods for a type 1 diabetes polygene (IDDM6) on chromosome 18q21. Hum. Mol Genet 6: 1003-10.

26. Morahan G, Huang D, Tait BD, et al (1996) Markers on distal chromosome 2q linked to insulin-dependent diabetes mellitus. Science 272:1811-3.

27. Nisticò L, Buzzetti R, Pritchard LE, et al (1996) The CTLA-4 gene region of chromosome 2q33 is linked to, and associated with, type 1 diabetes. Hum Mol Genet 5:1075-80.

28. O'Connor G, Neufeld DS, Greenberg DA, et al (1993) Lack of disease associated HLA-DQ restriction fragment length polymorphisms in families with autoimmune thyroid disease. Autoimmunity 14:237-41.

29. Payami H, Joe S, Thomson G (1989) Autoimmune thyroid disease in type 1 diabetic families. Genet Epidemiol 6:137-41.

30. Pearce SHS, Vaidya B, Imrie H, et al (1999) Further evidence for a susceptibility locus on chromosome 20q13.11 in families with

dominant transmission of Graves' disease. Am J Hum Genet 65:1462-5.

31. Risch N (1987) Assessing the role of HLA-linked and unlinked determinants of disease. Am J Hum Genet 40:1-14.

32. Roman SH, Greenberg D, Rubinstein P, et al (1992) Genetics of autoimmune thyroid disease: lack of evidence for linkage to HLA within families. J Clin Endocrinol Metab 74:496-503.

33. Shai R, Quismorio FP Jr, Li L, et al (1999) Genome-wide screen for systemic lupus erythematosus susceptibility genes in multiplex families. Hum Mol Genet 8:639-44.

34. Suarez BK, Hampe CL (1994) Linkage and association. Am J Hum Genet 54:554-9.

35. Tomer Y, Barbesino G, Keddache M, et al (1997) Mapping of a major susceptibility locus for Graves' disease (GD-1) to chromosome 14q31. J Clin Endocrinol Metab 82:1645-8.

36. Tomer Y, Barbesino G, Greenberg DA, et al (1998a) Linkage analysis of candidate genes in autoimmune thyroid disease. III. Detailed analysis of chromosome 14 localizes Graves' disease-1 (GD-1) close to multinodular goiter-1 (MNG-1). J Clin Endocrinol Metab 83:4321-7.

37. Tomer Y, Barbesino G, Greenberg DA, et al (1998b) A new Graves disease-susceptibility locus maps to chromosome 20q11.2. Am J Hum Genet 63:1749-56.

38. Tomer Y, Barbesino G, Greenberg DA, et al (1999) Mapping the Major Susceptibility Loci for Familial Graves' and Hashimoto's Diseases: Evidence for Genetic Heterogeneity and Gene Interactions. J Clin Endocrinol Metab 84:4656-64.

39. Tomer Y, Greenberg DA, Barbesino G, et al (2001) CTLA-4 and Not CD28 Is a Susceptibility Gene for Thyroid Autoantibody Production. J Clin Endocrinol Metab 86:1687-93.

40. Torfs CP, King MC, Huey B, et al (1986) Genetic interrelationship between insulin-dependent diabetes mellitus, the autoimmune thyroid diseases, and rheumatoid arthritis. Am J Hum Genet 38:170-87.

41. Tunbridge WGM, Evered DC, Hall R, et al (1977) The spectrum of thyroid disease in a community: the Whickham survey. Clin Endocrinol 7:481-93.

42. Vaidya B, Imrie H, Perros P, et al (1999a) The cytotoxic T lymphocyte antigen-4 is a major Graves' disease locus. Hum Mol Genet 8:1195-9.
43. Vaidya B, Imrie H, Perros P, et al (1999b) Cytotoxic T lymphocyte antigen-4 (CTLA-4) gene polymorphism confers susceptibility to thyroid associated orbitopathy. Lancet 354:743-4.
44. Vaidya B, Imrie H, Perros P, et al (2000) Evidence for a new Graves disease susceptibility locus at chromosome 18q21. Am J Hum Genet 66:1710-4.
45. Villanueva R, Inzerillo AM, Tomer Y, et al (2000) Limited genetic susceptibility to severe Graves' ophthalmopathy: no role for CTLA-4 but evidence for an environmental etiology. Thyroid 10:791-8.
46. Vyse TJ, Todd JA (1996) Genetic analysis of autoimmune disease. Cell 85:311-8.
47. Waterhouse P, Penninger JM, Timms E, et al (1995) Lymphoproliferative disorders with early lethality in mice deficient in Ctla-4. Science 270:985-8.
48. Yanagawa T, Mangklabruks A, Chang YB, et al (1993) Human histocompatability leukocyte antigen-DQA1*0501 allele associated with genetic susceptibility to Graves' disease in a Caucasian population. J Clin Endocrinol Metab 76:1569-74.
49. Yanagawa T, Hidaka Y, Guimaraes V, et al (1995) CTLA-4 gene polymorphism associated with Graves' disease in a Caucasian population. J Clin Endocrinol Metab 80:41-5.
50. Yanagawa T, Taniyama M, Enomoto S, et al (1997) CTLA4 gene polymorphism confers susceptibility to Graves' disease in Japanese. Thyroid 7:843-6.

Table 1. Prevalence of Graves' Disease (GD) and autoimmune hypothyroidism (AH) in first-degree relatives of GD probands (n=190)

Affected relatives	GD (%)	AH (%)
Sisters	9 (4.7)	10 (5.3)
Brothers		0
Mothers	16 (8.4)	23 (12.1)
Fathers	1 (0.5)	3 (1.6)
Daughters	0	1 (0.5)
Sons	1 (0.5)	0
Total	**33 (17.4)**	**37 (19.5)**

Table 2. Prevalence of non-thyroidal autoimmune disorders in first-degree relatives of Graves' disease probands (n=190)

Autoimmune disorders	Number of probands with affected first-degree relatives (%)	Estimated prevalence in general population (%)*
Type 1 diabetes mellitus	10 (5.3)	0.40
Rheumatoid arthritis	9 (4.7)	1.00
Pernicious anaemia	3 (1.8)	0.15
Multiple sclerosis	1 (0.5)	0.10
Ankylosing spondylitis	1 (0.5)	0.13

*References: Vyse & Todd, 1996; Jacobson et al., 1997.

Table 3. Intra-familial association between Graves' disease (GD) probands and unaffected sibcontrols at chromosome 2q31-q36 markers

Markers	Marker map (cM)	Allele (mu)	GD probands*	Unaffected sibs*	p value[†]
D2S2314	00.0	116	6/12	5/13	0.500
D2S152	09.0	228	14/12	7/19	**0.044**
D2S389	11.5	203	10/12	5/17	0.304
D2S117	17.2	206	8/10	3/15	0.219
CTLA-4(49)A/G	19.5	G	20/6	10/16	**0.005**
CTLA-4(AT)n	19.6	112[§]	14/4	7/11	**0.020**
D2S116	21.1	150	9/7	3/13	0.099
D2S2289	23.2	205	13/15	8/20	0.405
D2S155	28.0	169	10/10	9/11	0.500
D2S157	35.3	190	5/11	4/12	0.500
D2S137	41.4	149	15/11	5/21	**0.014**
D2S301	46.3	231	9/9	4/14	0.246
D2S120	51.6	187	16/10	9/17	0.142

*Number of occurrences of candidate alleles/ non-occurrences (Curtis, 1997). The total number of candidate alleles differentially occurring in the probands and the unaffected siblings were compared.

[†]Fisher's exact test. Three most common candidate alleles were tested for association and p values were corrected for multiple allelic comparisons, except for the markers D2S152, CTLA-4A/G and CTLA-4(AT)n, where candidate alleles were known.

[§]112 mu allele of CTLA-4(AT)n is equivalent to the 106 mu allele described by Yanagawa et al. (1995).

Table 4. Two-point linkage analysis at the various candidate loci in Graves' disease families

Locus	Chromosome	Marker	NPL	p value
IDDM4	11q13	*D11S1917*	-0.62	0.73
IDDM5	6q25	*ESR*	0.91	0.18
IDDM6	18q21	*D18S41*	1.57	0.06
IDDM8	6q27	*D6S281*	0.48	0.31
IDDM10	10p11-q11	*D10S193*	-1.05	0.85
FUT-2	19q13	*D19S888*	-0.85	0.80
AITD1	6p11	*D6S257*	1.23	0.11
SLE1	1q42	*D1S437*	-0.30	0.62
MS locus	17q23	*D17S795*	-0.69	0.75

Table 5. Linkage of Graves' disease to different chromosomal loci in different populations.

Chromosomal location	U.K. families (Newcastle)[*]	U.K. families (Birmingham)[#]	U.S.A. families[$]	Other linked autoimmune disorders[¶]
6p21 (*MHC*)	Yes	Yes	No	T1DM (*IDDM1*), SLE, MS, RA and others
2q33 (*CTLA-4*)	Yes	Yes	No°	T1DM (*IDDM12*), Coeliac, Crohn's disease
2q35	Weak	-	-	T1DM (*IDDM13*), RA
18q21	Yes	-	-	T1DM (*IDDM6*), RA, SLE, Crohn's disease
Xp11	Yes	-	-	T1DM (*IDDMX*), MS, RA
14q31 (*GD1*)	No	-	Yes	T1DM (*IDDM11*), SLE
20q13 (*GD2*)	Weak[†]	-	Yes	SLE
Xq21 (*GD3*)	No	-	Yes	-

[*]References: Pearce et al., 1999; Vaidya et al., 1999a, 2000; Imrie et al., 2001.
[#]References: Heward et al., 1998, 1999.
[$]References: Tomer et al., 1997, 1998a, 1998b, 1999; Barbesino et al.,1998.

¹Selected references: Davies et al., 1994; Nisticò et al., 1996; Morahan et al., 1996; Marron et al., 2000; Merriman et al., 1997; Cornelis et al., 1998; Cucca et al., 1998; Becker, 1999; Shai et al., 1999; Duerr et al., 2000.
†Linkage found only in the GD families with apparent dominant mode of transmission.

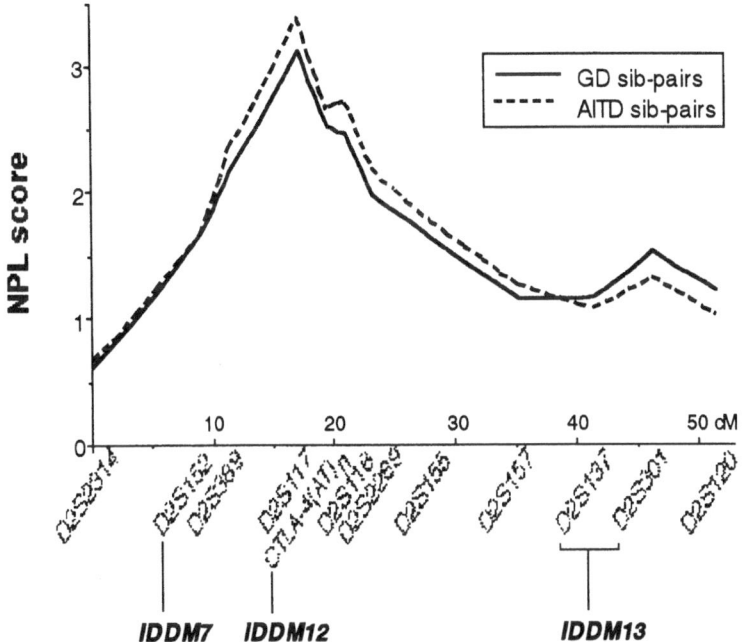

Figure 1. Multipoint linkage analysis of chromosome 2q31-q36. The NPL score obtained by scoring all affected subjects with GD (solid line) and AITD (dashed line) using the GENEHUNTER package is shown, against the marker map on the x-axis. The single nucleotide polymorphism *CTLA-4A/G* is at the same map position as *CTLA-4(AT)n*. The peak NPL of 3.43 occurs at the marker *D2S117* with a smaller separate peak (NPL 1.54) at *D2S301*.

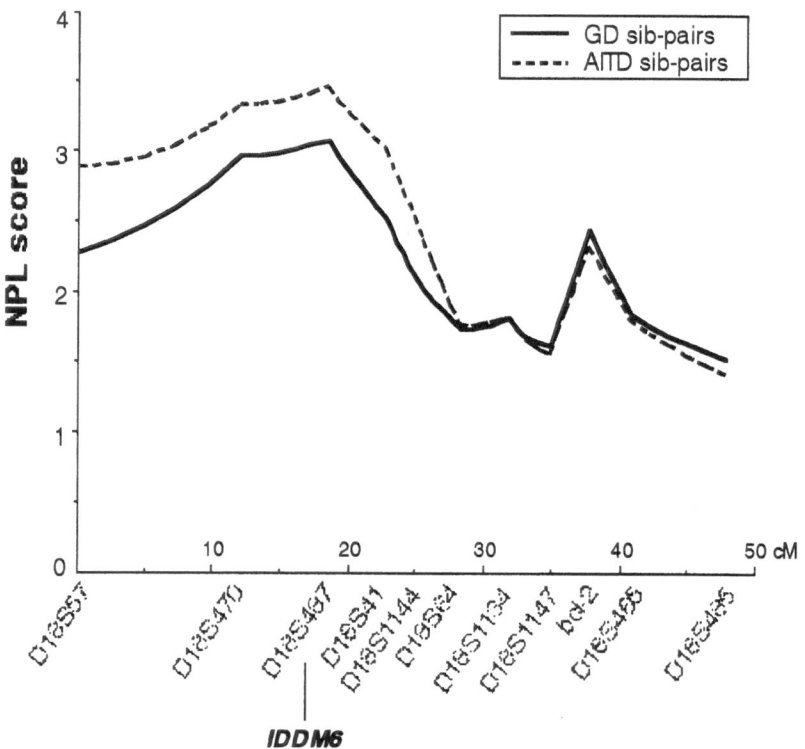

Figure 2. Multipoint linkage analysis of chromosome 18q12-q22. The NPL score obtained for GD (solid line) and AITD (dashed line) is shown, against the marker map on the x-axis. The peak NPL score of 3.46 occurs at the marker *D18S487*.

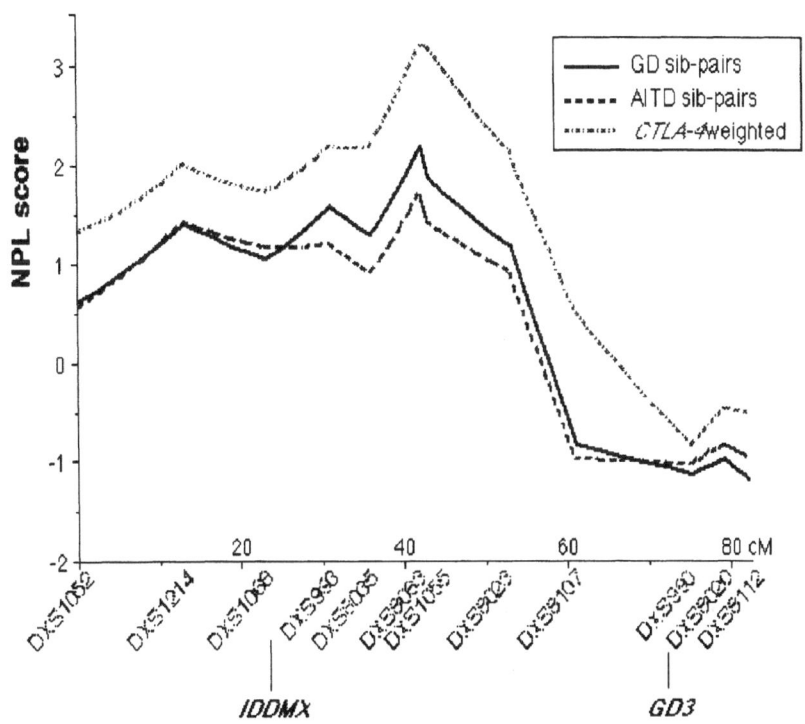

Figure 3. Multipoint linkage analysis of chromosome Xp13-q22. The NPL score obtained for GD (solid line) and AITD (dashed line) is shown, against the marker map on the x-axis. The NPL score of GD affected subjects when weighted (0 or 1) for allele sharing at the *CTLA-4* (*D2S117*) marker under an epistatic model is shown by the interrupted dash line. The peak unweighted NPL of 2.21 (p=0.014) occurs at the marker *DXS8083*. The peak *CTLA-4* weighted NPL of 3.18 (p=0.001) occurs 2cM away at *DXS1055*.

The involvement of the HLA region in genetic susceptibility to Graves' disease

Dr.J.M.Heward
Department of Medicine, University of Birmingham, Birmingham, UK

Key words
Graves' disease, autoimmune disease, HLA, DRB1*03, DQA1*0501

Graves' disease (GD) is an autoimmune disease of the thyroid gland characterized by hyperthyroidism, the presence of a diffuse goitre and in some cases ophthalmopathy and pretibial myxoedema. The frequency and severity of the symptoms, however, varies between individuals. The disease usually presents in the fourth decade of life (Vanderpump et al, 1995) and is reported to be 8 - 10 times more common in women than men (Wong et al, 1995) with the prevalence in females and males being around 20/1000 and 2/1000, respectively (Tunbridge et al, 1977). GD is a complex disorder thought to fit a multifactorial pattern of inheritance where disease develops due to an interaction between genetic components and environmental and endogenous factors (Stenszky et al, 1985). No single gene has been identified as causative for Graves' disease and many studies indicate that the involvement of multiple genes is necessary for the development of autoimmunity in this disease (Farid, 1992). Due to the incomplete penetrance of genetic components seen in Graves' disease it is reasonable to assume that other factors are influencing the development of disease in genetically susceptible individuals. These factors include infection, stress, synthetic chemicals and iodine.

Serological evidence for recent bacterial or viral infections has been reported in 36% of newly diagnosed patients with Graves' disease and only 10% of control subjects (Valtonen et al, 1986). The leading candidate as an infective trigger for Graves' disease is *Yersinia enterocolitica*. This is primarily known to cause food poisoning but studies of patients with Graves' disease have shown that large numbers carry antibodies to *Yersinia* antigen (Shenkman and Bottone, 1976) and that many *Yersinia* antibodies cross-react with thyroid antigens with differing affinity. Antibodies to plasmid-encoded release proteins of *Yersinia enterocolitica* have been found in 72% of patients with Graves' disease, 81% of patients with recurrent disease but also in 35% control subjects (Wenzel *et al*, 1988). It has also been demonstrated that *Yersinia* has a saturable binding site for TSH (Weiss *et al*, 1983). Animal studies in rats have demonstrated induction of lymphocytic thyroiditis after immunization with *Yersinia enterocolitica* purified outer membrane protein (Ebner *et al*, 1991). Despite these findings there is a lack of evidence that infection with *Yersinia* leads directly or indirectly to autoimmune thyroid disease in humans as most patients with *Yersinia* infection do not develop Graves' disease (Toivanen and Toivanen, 1994). Retroviruses have also been implicated in the aetiology of Graves' disease. A recent study reported the presence of antibodies against a human intracisternal type A retroviral particle (HIAP) in over 85% of patients with Graves' disease but a complete absence of antibodies in age and gender matched control subjects. Upon further examination in families with a high incidence of Graves' disease it was noted that there was a highly significant association between HIAP antibody positivity, HLA susceptibility and Graves' disease thus indicating that pathogenesis of Graves' disease, at least in these families, may be due to interaction between the immune response to HIAP and genetic susceptibility provided by the HLA region (Jaspan *et al*, 1996). Further studies will be required to ascertain whether people at risk of Graves' disease may be identified by these criteria.

Stress has long since been implicated in the aetiology of Graves' disease with population based case control studies demonstrating that patients presenting with Graves' disease have experienced very stressful episodes in the few months prior to diagnosis (Kung, 1995). The mechanism by which this occurs is unclear but may be related to changes in the hypothalmic-pituitary-adrenal axis that occur during stressful events which in turn may lead to suppression of immune function (Fricchione and Stefano, 1994). However, presentation of clinical disease is a poor marker for early immune events that occur in the pathogenesis of Graves' disease, therefore, recent stressful events may have occurred after initiation of the disease process but may have exacerbated clinical presentation (McIver and Morris, 1998).

Synthetic chemicals can be released into the environment as pesticides or by industrial activity. The role that these chemicals play in disruption of thyroid function and development of disease is controversial as few studies have been performed in humans (Brucker-Davis, 1998). Observations of wildlife in polluted areas clearly show a significant incidence of goitre and thyroid dysfunction (Moccia *et al*, 1981). However, studies in adult humans have indicated that background levels of chemicals do not affect thyroid function although higher levels may produce mild thyroid dysfunction (Brucker-Davis, 1998). Few studies have been performed on the effect that these chemicals may have on *in utero* development or childhood thyroid function. Several preliminary studies indicate that neurological function is impaired in children who have been exposed to high levels of polychlorinated biphenyls and dioxins (Jacobson and Jacobson, 1996) but it is unclear if this is caused by thyroid disruption *in utero* or by neurotoxicity after birth. It is clear that further studies are needed to clarify this issue.

Animal studies have indicated that iodine intake and exposure are important factors in the development of experimental thyroid disease (McIver and Morris, 1998). Rats that are genetically susceptible to thyroiditis develop disease more often when iodine is supplemented into their diet than when it is withheld (Allen *et al*, 1986). Data to support these mechanisms in human Graves' disease is lacking. It appears that in areas with a sufficient iodine concentration, iodine does not play a significant role in the pathogenesis of Graves' disease (McIver and Morris, 1998).

Although these environmental agents may aid in triggering presentation of GD strong evidence exists that the underlying basis of the disease is genetic with evidence supporting this being provided by looking at disease clustering within families and concordance rates in both monozygotic (MZ) and dizygotic (DZ) twins.

Family studies are valuable not only to provide evidence for clustering of a particular disease within a family but also to ascertain whether certain autoimmune diseases cluster together in individual families. It has long since been noted by clinicians that autoimmune thyroid disease is frequently seen in patients with type 1 diabetes. This has been confirmed by the 5th Genetic Analysis Workshop with the finding of at least one case of autoimmune thyroid disease in 40% of type 1 diabetic families (Payami *et al*, 1989), a result supported by data from the British Diabetic Association Warren Repository where 22% of type 1 diabetic families had at least one case of autoimmune thyroid disease (S.C.Bain, personal communication). These results indicate

the importance of a family resource in the ascertainment of genetic susceptibility, not only to Graves' disease, but to other autoimmune diseases that may
have a shared genetic basis. Family data are also important as, not only do the
members share genes, they may also share the same environment thus leading
to the same exposure to environmental stimulation that may affect the disease
process. A family history of Graves' disease is found in about 50% of patients
with this disorder (Bartels, 1941). Studies in families with Graves' disease
have indicated that disease occurs in about 1% of the probands first degree
male relatives and 5% of their first degree female relatives thus enabling the
λs for Graves' disease to be estimated at 7.5 - 10 (Allahabadia and Gough,
1999).

Twin studies are also an invaluable tool in developing understanding
of susceptibility to autoimmune disease. This resource can aid understanding
as to the scale of contribution to susceptibility to disease of genetic and environmental components by looking at monozygotic and dizygotic twins. As
monozygotic twins share an identical genetic makeup, higher concordance
rates in these twins when compared with dizygotic twins would be expected if
genetic components are involved in the disease process. In the absence of a
genetic basis, it would be reasonable to presume that both types of twins
would have a similar concordance rate. Early studies of both MZ and DZ
twins indicated high concordance rates (86% MZ vs 40% DZ and 64% MZ vs
6% DZ) in both types of twin. However, upon further examination of these
data it must be noted that these early studies did not distinguish between
autoimmune and nonautoimmune hyperthyroidism and some even included
patients with simple nontoxic goitre, thus rendering these results difficult to
interpret (Harvald and Hauge, 1956; Verschuer, 1958). A more recent study in
Danish twins, where strict criteria were applied for the diagnosis of Graves'
disease, indicated much lower concordance rates (36% MZ vs 0% DZ) (Brix *et
al*, 1998). These rates were still significantly higher in MZ twins confirming
that genetic factors do play a role in the aetiology of Graves' disease. The
concordance rate still falls far short of 100%, however, indicating that non-
genetic factors must play a role in the development of Graves' disease.

As mentioned previously, GD is a polygenic disorder with a number of
genes contributing to overall susceptibility. Candidate gene studies suggest
that both the HLA region on chromosome 6p21 and the CTLA-4 gene region
on chromosome 2q33 both contribute to disease susceptibility. Genome wide
searches have implicated 3 further regions on chromosome 14(GD1) (Tomer *et*

al, 1997), chromosome 20 (GD2) (Tomer *et al*, 1998) and the X chromosome(GD3) (Barbesino *et al*, 1998). The HLA region on chromosome 6p21 has been the focus of many studies and will be the topic of this review highlighting why it may play a role in susceptibility to GD and on studies that have been performed on this region.

The HLA genes are located in the major histocompatibility complex (MHC) on the short arm of chromosome 6 (6p21). The MHC can be divided into three regions:-class I, class II and class III (Figure1) which span about 4 million base pairs and contain many genes.

The class I region is located at the telomeric end of the MHC. It contains the HLA-A, HLA-B and HLA-C genes which code for the α peptide chains of the HLA-A, -B and -C transplantation antigens. Class I molecules are expressed on the cell surface of nucleated cells and are involved in the presentation of peptides, such as viral antigens, to cytotoxic (CD8 positive) T cells.

The class II region contains many genes that are involved in antigen processing and presentation. At the telomeric end of the region are the DR and DQ genes which code for the α and β peptide chains of the HLA class II molecules. Class II molecules are also membrane bound proteins which are expressed on the cell surface of B-lymphocytes, macrophages, dendritic cells and activated T lymphocytes. They are involved in presentation of intracellularly processed antigens to CD4-positive helper T cells. The genes that encode proteins involved in antigen processing lie centrally within the class II region. These genes include the large multifunctional proteasome genes (LMP 2 and 7) and the transporter associated with antigen processing genes (TAP 1 and 2). LMP 2 and 7 are involved in the degradation and cleavage of antigenic peptide in the cytosol before the TAP proteins can transport the peptide into the lumen of the endoplasmic reticulum (ER). The DM genes lie next to the LMP and TAP genes in the class II region.   HLA-DM is involved in the loading of antigenic peptides onto class II molecules. The DP genes are the most centromeric in the class II region. DPA1 and B1 code for the α and β peptide chains that make up the class II molecule. They are structurally and functionally similar to HLA-DR and -DQ and are involved in the presentation of antigen to CD4 positive T cells.

The class III region is located between the class I and II regions and containsgenes involved in the complement system (C2, C4 and Bf), the heat shock protein (HSP70) genes and the tumour necrosis factor (TNF) genes.

Almost all of the studies examining the HLA region and Graves' disease have been performed using population based case control datasets. Early studies looking at association of the class I region with Graves' disease observed an association with HLA-B8 in populations from Canada (Farid *et al*,1976), the UK (Mather *et al*, 1980) and Black Africans from South Africa (Kalk *et al*, 1983). Most subsequent studies have confirmed this association and attention has tended to be more focussed on the effect that the HLA class II region genes have on genetic susceptibility to Graves' disease.

The HLA class II genes aid in antigen presentation to CD4 positive T cells. In particular the DRB, DQA1 and DQB1 genes are highly polymorphic which results in a potentially large number of functional HLA molecules which would be able to present a large number of foreign antigens. These molecules play a major role in maintaining tolerance to self antigens, thus a breakdown in this tolerance may lead to the development of autoimmune diseases such as GD. The fact that aberrant expression of HLA class II antigens is seen on follicular cells (the target cells in GD) and on activated lymphocytes in patients with GD make this region an ideal candidate for involvement in the genetic susceptibility to GD.

Early population based case control studies of the HLA class II DR genes found a strong association with HLA-DR3 in Canadian (Farid *et al*, 1979), French (Allanic *et al*, 1980), Swedish (Dahlberg *et al*, 1981) and German (Boehm *et al*, 1992) populations. The French and Swedish studies, however, reported no association between the increase in DR3 and different manifestations of the disease, such as goitre or ophthalmopathy, or the severity of clinical and biochemical signs. Despite this strong association of DR3 with disease in the above populations it was noted that DR3 was decreased in frequency in Sardinian patients with Graves' disease (Boehm *et al*, 1992) and disease association in the Japanese appeared to be almost exclusively due to class I molecules (Ito *et al*, 1989). From these results it seems clear that, in most populations, DR3 plays an important role in genetic susceptibility to Graves' disease but also that other susceptibility loci are involved.

Further population based case control studies into the role of the HLA class II genes have implicated the DQ allele, DQA1*0501, in genetic susceptibility to Graves' disease. A study by Yanagawa *et al;*1993 found a significant increase in frequency of DQA1*0501 in Caucasian patients with Graves' disease when compared with control subjects. There was also an observed increase in DR3, which is in tight LD with DQA1*0501, although this did not remain significant after correction of the p value. No observed increase was seen in any

DQB1 alleles. Interestingly, it was noted that, upon exclusion of DR3-positive patients, DQA1*0501 was still significantly associated with disease, suggesting that this locus may be the primary aetiological determinant for Graves' disease within the MHC region. The association of DQA1*0501 with Graves' disease has since been replicated by Badenhoop *et al;*1995 and Barlow *et al;*1996. However, the former study only examined the frequencies of HLA-DQ alleles, thus making it impossible to ascertain whether an independent effect of DQA1*0501 was seen over and above that seen with DR3. The study by Barlow *et al;* also found an increase in frequency of DQA1*0501 over and above linkage disequilibrium with DR3, thus seeming to confirm the findings of Yanagawa *et al;*. However, this study did not correct the p values for the number of alleles seen. Correction of p values in this study would have rendered the result nonsignificant. These studies may differ due to genuine racial and geographical differences in the populations used, however, it must be noted that sample size in these populations was relatively small which may account for the differences observed.

A small number of family based studies have been performed but none have replicated, with linkage analysis, the findings of the population based case control studies. This is almost certainly due to the use of too few families within the dataset (between 300 and 2,500 affected sib pair families and between 100 and 340 simplex families are needed), thus the dataset lacks the power to detect linkage. Very early studies were performed using just one or two families to attempt to further elucidate the role played by the HLA genes in Graves' disease. A more recent study, using lod score analysis, failed to find any linkage to HLA in families with Graves' disease (Tomer *et al*,1997). However Vaidya *et al*, 1999 performed a study on affected sibpairs using 5 markers spanning the MHC on chromosome 6p21. Using non parametric analysis, linkage was observed at this locus with a peak NPL score of 1.95 between the markers D6S273 and TNFα. These results were observed in a UK dataset and therefore the different results observed may be due to genuine geographical and racial differences and also due to the statistical methods employed for analysis.

From these previous studies it seems obvious that DRB1*03 and DQA1*0501 are involved in genetic susceptibility to GD in certain populations. However, lack of replication in many family based datasets could be seen as evidence that these results were spurious due to the relatively small number of subjects used in each study. It has been noted in Type 1 diabetes that the HLA region has a λs of 1.2-1.5 and in order to detect this effect at least 500-600 affected sib pairs are needed, therefore, it may be construed that this lack of replication is due to insufficient numbers within the family based datasets used.

In order to verify the associations of these genes with Graves' disease we undertook a study within our laboratory to genotype the HLA class II genes, DRB1, DQB1 and DQA1 in a large ethnically homogeneous population based case control dataset. A second large family based dataset was then used to replicate the findings of the case control dataset and exclude population stratification by using the transmission disequilibrium test (TDT). To date 478 patients with GD, 425 control subjects and 210 families have been genotyped for the aforementioned HLA genes.

A strong association of the alleles DRB1*03 and DQA1*0501 with GD was observed in the case control dataset (Table 1). Both alleles were significantly associated with disease after correction of the p values for the number of alleles tested (**DRB1*03**: GD 45% vs control subjects 27.3%; $\chi^2 = 39.4$; pc = 1.4 x 10^{-5}; odds ratio = 2.45; 95% confidence limits = 1.84-3.25; **DQA1*0501**: GD 61.3% vs control subjects 41.2%; $\chi^2 = 36.5$; pc = 7 x 10^{-6}; odds ratio (OR) = 2.26; 95% confidence limits (CL) = 1.73-2.95). Due to the tight linkage disequilibrium between DRB1*03, DQB1*02 and DQA1*0501, distribution of the haplotype DRB1*03-DQB1*02-DQA1*0501 was compared between patients with Graves' disease and control subjects (Table 1). A significant increase in frequency of this haplotype was seen in patients with Graves' disease when compared with control subjects (44.7% vs 24.2%, respectively; $\chi^2 = 41.6$; pc = 1 x 10^{-6} OR = 2.52; 95% CL = 1.89 – 3.35).

Due to recent reports of the independent association of DQA1*0501 with Graves' disease, this allele was compared in DRB1*03 negative patients with Graves' disease and control subjects (Table 2), in order to determine whether DQA1*0501 was independently associated with Graves' disease in our dataset. No independent association of this allele was seen in DRB1*03 negative patients with Graves' disease when compared with DRB1*03 negative control subjects (29.7% vs 22.6%, respectively; $\chi^2 = 3.78$; p = 0.052).

In order to replicate the finding of the population based case control dataset, transmission of the haplotype DRB1*03-DQB1*02-DQA1*0501 from heterozygous parents to affected and unaffected siblings was analyzed using the TDT. Of the 210 families available for study, 115 were informative for this haplotype. Transmission data is summarized in Table 3. A significant increase in transmission (T) compared to nontransmission (NT) of the DRB1*03-DQB1*02-DQA1*0501 haplotype was seen in affected offspring [89T (68.4%) vs 41NT (31.6%); χ^2 = 17.72; p = 1 x 10^{-4}]. There was no preferential transmission of this haplotype to unaffected offspring [49T (44.9%) vs 60NT (55.1%); χ^2 = 1.11; p = ns]. The 2 x 2 test of heterogeneity comparing transmission of the DRB1*03-DQB1*02-DQA1*0501 haplotype to affected and unaffected offspring confirmed that the significant excess of transmissions to affected offspring was not the result of segregation distortion (χ^2 = 13.95; p = 5 x 10^{-4}). These results strongly suggest that the HLA region does play a major role in the genetic susceptibility to GD and emphasises the importance of large datasets when attempting to draw meaningful conclusions from these type of studies.

Although from this study the HLA region is clearly involved in the genetic susceptibility to the development of GD, probably contributing around 25% in the UK, other genes must also be involved. Other immune response genes such as LMP2 and 7 have been excluded as conferring susceptibility to GD (Heward *et al*, 1999) but other genes such as the interleukins and TNF genes need to be further investigated in order to elucidate their role in genetic susceptibility to GD.

In conclusion, whilst the exact mechanism of action of these genes is unknown, there is increasing evidence to suggest that polymorphism of genes involved in the presentation of autoantigen/antigen to the T cell receptor such as the MHC-HLA class II molecules are likely to play a pivotal role in the development of GD. Functional studies of these molecules and pathways are crucial in order to understand the mechanism by which GD is caused.

Acknowledgements

I would like to acknowledge Dr.S.C.L.Gough, Professor J.Franklyn, Dr.A.Allahabadia, Jackie Carr-Smith, Angela Daly, Jacquie Daykin, Dr.R.Nithiyananthan and Sarah Gibson who have been involved in this work in Birmingham and also the Wellcome Trust for supporting this work.

References

1. Allahabadia A. and Gough S.C.L (1999) The different approaches to the genetic analysis of autoimmune thyroid disease. *Journal of Endocrinology* 163:7-13.
2. Allanic H., Fauchet R., Lorcy Y., Heim J., Gueguen M., Leguerrier A.M. and Genetet B (1980) HLA and Graves' disease: an association with HLA-DRw3. *J Clin Endocrinol Metab* 51: 863-867.
3. Allen E.M., Appel M.C. and Braverman L.E (1986) The effect of iodide ingestion on the development of spontaneous lymphocytic thyroiditis in the diabetes-prone BB/W rat. *Endocrinology* 118: 1977-1981.
4. Badenhoop K., Walfish P.G., Rau H., Fischer S., Nicolay A., Bogner U., Schleusener H. and Usadel K.H (1995) Susceptibility and resistance alleles of human leukocyte antigen (HLA) DQA1 and HLA DQB1 are shared in endocrine autoimmune disease. *J Clin Endocrinol Metab* 80: 2112-2117.
5. Barbesino G., Tomer Y., Concepcion E.S., Davies T.F. and Greenberg D.A (1998) Linkage analysis of candidate genes in autoimmune thyroid disease. II. Selected gender-related genes and the X-chromosome. International Consortium for the Genetics of Autoimmune Thyroid Disease. *J Clin Endocrinol Metab* 83: 3290-3295.
6. Barlow A.B., Wheatcroft N., Watson P. and Weetman A.P (1996) Association of HLA-DQA1*0501 with Graves' disease in English Caucasian men and women. *Clin Endocrinol (Oxf)* 44,: 73-77.
7. Bartels E.D (1941) Heredity in Graves' disease. With remarks on heredity in toxic adenoma in the thyroid, non-toxic goitre, and myxoedema (thesis). Copenhagen: Einar Munksgaard, pp.3-384.
8. Boehm B.O., Thomas H., Lee J., Chan S.H., Cheah J.S., Nishimura Y., Dong R.P., Sasazuki T., Contu L., Carcassi C. and Zaretskaya Y (1992) Graves' disease study. *Disease components* W6.3: 710-713.
9. Brix T.H., Christensen K., Holm N.V., Harvald B. and Hegedus L (1998) A population-based study of Graves' disease in Danish twins. *Clin Endocrinol (Oxf)* 48: 397-400.
10. Brucker-Davis F (1998) Effects of environmental synthetic chemicals on thyroid function. *Thyroid* 8: 827-856.
11. Dahlberg P A., Holmlund G., Karlsson F.A. and Safwenberg J (1981) HLA-A, -B, -C and -DR antigens in patients with Graves' disease and

their correlation with signs and clinical course. *Acta Endocrinol (Copenh)* 97: 42-47.

12. Ebner S., Alex S. and Klugman T (1991) Immunization with *Yersinia enterolitica* purified outer membrane protein induces lymphocytic thyroiditis in the BB/WOR rat.*Thyroid* 1 (supplement):S-28.

13. Farid N.R., Barnard J.M. and Marshall W.H (1976) The association of HLA with autoimmune thyroid disease in Newfoundland. The influence of HLA homozygosity in Graves' disease. *Tissue Antigens* 8: 181-189.

14. Farid N.R., Sampson L., Noel E.P., Barnard J.M., Mandeville R., Larsen B., Marshall W.H. and Carter N.D (1979) A study of human leukocyte D locus related antigens in Graves' disease. *J Clin Invest* 63,: 108-113.

15. Farid N.R (1992) Understanding the genetics of autoimmune thyroid disease--still an illusive goal!. *J Clin Endocrinol Metab* 74: 495A-495B.

16. Fricchione G.L. and Stefano G.B (1994) The stress response and auto-immunoregulation. *Adv Neuroimmunol* 4: 13-27.

17. Harvald B. and Hauge M (1956) A catemnistic investigation of Danish twins - A preliminary report. *Dan Med Bull* 3: 150-158.

18. Heward J.M., Allahabadia A., Sheppard M.C., Barnett A.H., Franklyn J.A. and Gough S.C.L (1999) Association of the large multifunctional proteasome (LMP2) gene with Graves' disease is a result of linkage disequilibrium with the HLA haplotype DRB1*0304-DQB1*02-DQA1*0501. *Clin End* 51: 115-118.

19. Ito M., Tanimoto M., Kamura H., Yoneda M., Morishima Y., Yamauchi K., Itatsu T., Takatsuki K. and Saito H (1989) Association of HLA antigen and restriction fragment length polymorphism of T cell receptor beta-chain gene with Graves' disease and Hashimoto's thyroiditis. *J Clin Endocrinol Metab* 69: 100-104.

20. Jacobson J.L. and Jacobson S.W (1996) Intellectual impairment in children exposed to polychlorinated biphenyls in utero. *N Engl J Med* 335: 783-789.

21. Jaspan J.B., Sullivan K., Garry R.F., Lopez M., Wolfe M., Clejan S., Yan C., Tenenbaum S., Sander D.M., Ahmed B. and Bryer-Ash M (1996) The interaction of a type A retroviral particle and class II human leukocyte antigen susceptibility genes in the pathogenesis of Graves' disease. *J Clin Endocrinol Metab* 81: 2271-2279.

22. Kalk W.J., Maier G., van Drimellen M., LevinJ. and Reinach S.G (1983) HLA antigens and Graves' disease in Black South Africans. *Tissue Antigens* 22: 7-15.

23. Kung A.W (1995) Life events, daily stresses and coping in patients with Graves' disease. *Clin Endocrinol (Oxf)* 42: 303-308.

24. Mather B.A., Roberts D.F., Scanlon M.F., Mukhtar E.D., Davies T.F., Smith B.R. and Hall R (1980) HLA antigens and thyroid autoantibodies in patients with Graves' disease and their first degree relatives. *Clin Endocrinol (Oxf)* 12: 155-163.

25. McIver B. and Morris J.C (1998) The pathogenesis of Graves' disease. In *Endocrinology and Metabolism Clinics of Nrth America*, 27:73-89.

26. Moccia R.D.,. Leatherland J.F. and Sonstegard R.A (1981) Quantitative interlake comparison of thyroid pathology in Great Lakes coho (Oncorhynchus kisutch) and chinook (Oncorhynchus tschawytscha) salmon. *Cancer Res* 41: 2200-2210.

27. Payami H., Joe S. and Thomson G (1989) Autoimmune thyroid disease in type I diabetic families. *Genet Epidemiol* 6: 137-141.

28. Shenkman L. and Bottone E.J (1976) Antibodies to Yersinia enterocolitica in thyroid disease. *Ann Intern Med* 85,: 735-739.

29. Stenszky V., Kozma L., Balazs C., Rochlitz S., Bear J.C. and Farid N.R (1985) The genetics of Graves' disease: HLA and disease susceptibility. *J Clin Endocrinol Metab* 61: 735-740.

30. Toivanen P. and Toivanen A (1994) Does Yersinia induce autoimmunity? *Int Arch Allergy Immunol* 104: 107-111.

31. Tomer Y., Barbesino G., Keddache M., Greenberg D.A. and Davies T.F (1997) Mapping of a major susceptibility locus for Graves' disease (GD-1) to chromosome 14q31. *J Clin Endocrinol Metab* 82: 1645-1648.

32. Tomer Y., Barbesino G., Greenberg D.A., Concepcion E. and Davies T.F (1998) A New Graves Disease-Susceptibility Locus Maps To Chromosome 20q11.2. *Am J Hum Genet* 63,: 1749-1756.

33. Tunbridge W.M.G., Evered D.C., Hall R., Appleton D., Brewis M., Clark F., Grimley Evans J., Young F., Bird T. and Smith P.A (1977) The spectrum of thyroid disease in a community: The Whickham Survey. *Clin Endocrinol* 7: 481-493.

34. Vaidya B., Imrie H., Perros P., Young E.T., Kelly W.F., Carr D., Large D.M., Toft A.D., McCarthy M.I., Kendall-Taylor P. and Pearce S.H (1999) The cytotoxic T lymphocyte antigen-4 is a major Graves' disease locus. *Hum Mol Genet* 8: 1195-1199.

35. Valtonen V.V., Ruutu P., Varis K., Ranki M., Malkamaki M. and Makela P.H (1986) Serological evidence for the role of bacterial infections in the pathogenesis of thyroid diseases. *Acta Med Scand* 219: 105-111.

36. Vanderpump M.P., Tunbridge W.M., French J.M., Appleton D., Bates D., Clark F., Grimley Evans J., Hasan D.M., Rodgers H. and Tunbridge F (1995) The incidence of thyroid disorders in the community: a twenty-year follow-up of the Whickham Survey. *Clin Endocrinol (Oxf)* 43: 55-68.

37. Verschuer O.V (1958) Die zwillingforschung im dienste der inneren medizin. *Verh dtsch Ges inn Med* 64: 262-273.

38. Weiss M., Ingbar S.H., Winblad S. and Kasper D (1983) Demonstration of a saturable binding site for thyrotropin in Yersinia enterocolitica. *Science* 219: 1331-1333.

39. Wenzel B.E., Heesemann J., Wenzel K.W. and Scriba P.C (1988) Antibodies to plasmid-encoded proteins of enteropathogenic Yersinia in patients with autoimmune thyroid disease. *Lancet* 1: 56.

40. Wong G.W., Kwok M.Y. and Ou Y (1995) High incidence of juvenile Graves' disease in Hong Kong. *Clin Endocrinol (Oxf)* 43: 697-700.

41. Yanagawa T., Mangklabruks A., Chang Y.B., Okamoto Y., Fisfalen M.E., Curran P.G. and DeGroot L.J (1993) Human histocompatibility leukocyte antigen-DQA1*0501 allele associated with genetic susceptibility to Graves' disease in a Caucasian population. *J Clin Endocrinol Metab* 76: 1569-1574.

HLA and Autoimmune Thyroid Diseases

Ken Yamamoto and Takehiko Sasazuki
Medical Institute of Bioregulation, Kyushu University,
Maidashi 3-1-1, Higashi-ku, Fukuoka, 812-8582, Japan
Tel: 81 92 642 6827 Fax: 81 92 632 0150
e-mail: sasazuki@bioreg.kyushu-u.ac.jp

Introduction

Autoimmune thyroid diseases (AITD) including Graves disease (GD) and Hashimoto thyroiditis (HT) are typical organ-specific autoimmune diseases and genetic factors are suggested to be involved in their pathogenesis, based on the existence of multiplex families and the difference in concordant rate of the disease between monozygotic and dizygotic twins (1-3). In addition, there exist families with both GD and HT, and cases in which GD evolves into HT, suggesting common and disease-specific genetic factors controlling the susceptibility to the diseases. The major histocompatibility complex (MHC) has been shown to control both immune responsiveness to natural antigens and susceptibility to some diseases in humans and in experimental animals (4, 5), and the association between AITD and human MHC (HLA) has been reported in various ethnic groups (6-10). In this report we will identified the differences and similarity in immunogenetic features between GD and HT based on the analysis of HLA at both DNA and serological levels in Japanese.

Key Words

Graves' disease, autoimmune thyroid disease, Hashimoto's thyroiditis, HLA, HLA-A2, HLA–DPB1*0501, HLA–DRB1*0303, peptide

Functional features of HLA

HLA molecules are highly polymorphic glycoproteins. HLA class I molecules, HLA-A, -B and -C, are expressed on nucleated cells and class II molecules, HLA-DR, -DQ and –DP, are essentially expressed on thymic epithelial cells and antigen presenting cells (APCs) such as dendritic cells, macrophages, and B cells. According to polymorphism at the peptide-binding groove, these molecules present distinct sets of self or foreign antigenic peptides for the recognition by TCRs expressed on CD8$^+$ or CD4$^+$ T cells. HLA molecules are shown to be critical in the differentiation of CD4$^+$CD8$^+$ immature thymocytes into CD4$^-$CD8$^+$ or CD4$^+$CD8$^-$ mature thymocytes that elicit immune response to foreign antigenic peptides bound to self-HLA molecules in the periphery. Because HLA is highly polymorphic and T cell repertoire is shaped by HLA/peptide complex in the thymus, immune responsiveness to a given antigenic peptide in the periphery may be pre-determined. Focusing on the events in the periphery, the interaction of HLA/peptide/TCR complex introduces activation of T cells with secretion of several cytokines, some of which subsequently help maturation of B cells to antibody-secreting plasma cells. In addition, the functional maturation of CD8$^+$ T cells to cytotoxic CD8$^+$ T cells requires cell-cell contacts between activated CD4$^+$ T cells and APCs through the interaction of CD40 with CD40-L. Thus, presentation of antigenic peptides by HLA class II molecules may play an important role in determining the quality and the quantity of immune response in the periphery.

HLA-linked genetic factors involved in the pathogenesis of AITD

HLA and Graves disease in Japanese

The frequencies of HLA-A2, -B46 and –Cw11 were increased in GD patients. The increased frequency of HLA-B46 is consistent with the other reports (7, 11), but we could not confirm the increased frequencies of HLA-A11, -B5, -B35, and –B46 in GD patients. No positive association was observed with HLA-DR or –DQ antigens as was previously reported (11). On the other hand, frequencies of HLA-A24, -B7, -B52, and –DR1 were decreased in GD patients. Because A24, B7, and DR1, and A24 and B52, respectively, are in linkage disequilibria in the Japanese population (12), the A24-B7-DR1 and A24-B52 haplotypes might confer resistance to GD. When the p value was corrected by multiplying the number of tested alleles, only the association of HLA-A2 remained statistically significant (pc<0.02). In addition HLA-

DPB1*0501 was shown to be strongly associated with GD (pc<0.002). Because HLA-A2, -B46 and –Cw11 are known to be in linkage disequilibria, these results suggest that HLA-A2 and –DPB1*0501 are primarily associated with GD (13).

HLA and Hashimoto thyroiditis in Japanese

The frequencies of HLA-A2, -DRB4*0101, -DRB1*0403, -DQA1*03, -DQB1*0303 were significantly increased in HT patients. Among these associated alleles, DRB4*0101 showed strongest association with HT. Because HLA-DRB1*0403, -DQA1*03, and -DQB1*0303 are known to be in linkage disequilibria with –DRB4*0101 in Japanese population (12), their increased frequencies may reflect the linkage disequilibrium with –DRB4*0101. On the other hand, increased frequency of HLA-A2 in HT could not be explained by the linkage disequilibrium with –DRB4*0101, because no significant linkage disequilibrium between these alleles was found in the Japanese population. HLA-A2 is instead in linkage disequilibrium with the –B46-DR8-DQ6 haplotype, forming the HLA-A2-B46-DR8-DQ6 haplotype, in the Japanese population. The frequency of this haplotype was increased in the patients compared with that in controls. Thus, these results suggest that HLA-A2 and –DRB4*0101(-DR53) are primarily associated with HT (14).

Association of AITD with combination of HLA-A2 and HLA class II

Because both HLA-A2 and –DPB1*0501 are associated with GD, we investigated which factors was primarily associated with the disease by calculating the OR for risk to develop the disease in individuals positive for the associated HLA alleles. The highest OR was observed in individuals positive for both HLA-A2 and –DPB1*0501 (OR = 10.5), whereas –A2-positive –DPB1*0501-negative or –A2-negative –DPB1*0501-positive individuals exhibited an OR of 2.2 or 4.4, respectively (Table 1). This observation suggests that the combination of A2 and DPB1*0501 confers the susceptibility to GD. It is interesting that similar result was obtained in the analysis for HT. The highest OR was observed in individuals positive for HLA-A2 and –DRB4*0101 (OR = 12.8), whereas –A2-positive –DRB4*0101-negative or –A2-negative – DRB4*0101-positive individuals exhibited an OR of 7.3 or 7.5, respectively (Table 1). Theses results suggest that the susceptibility to AITD is controlled by multiple genes (class I and class II) in the HLA region (13, 14).

Table 1. High risk for AITD in individuals positive for both HLA-A2 and associated HLA class II

HLA-A2	DPB1*0501	Control[a] n=(317)	Graves[a] (n=76)	OR[b]
-	-	84	4	-
+	-	38	4	2.2
-	+	101	21	4.4
+	+	94	47	10.5

HLA-A2	DRB4*0101	Control[a] (n=317)	Hashimoto[a] (n=71)	OR[b]
-	-	67	2	-
+	-	46	10	7.3
-	+	120	27	7.5
+	+	84	32	12.8

a Individuals who have (+) or do not have (-) the HLA alleles are counted.
b ORs were calculated using the group of individuals who were negaive for both A2 and class II as a reference.

HLA-A2 subtypes and AITD

It is of interest that HLA-A2 is associated with both GD and HT. Our next study was to determine which A2 subtype is associated with these diseases. The DNA typing for HLA-A revealed that HLA-A*0201, -A*0206 and –A*0207 are common in Japanese population. As shown in Table 2, the frequency of HLA-A*0206 was increased in GD (the frequency in control versus that in GD, 15.3 % vs 32.2 %, RR = 2.63, p < 0.0005). On the other hand, interestingly, HLA-A*0207 but not -A*0206 was increased in HT (the frequency in control versus that in GD, 7.2 % vs 17.0 %, RR = 2.66, p < 0.005). We calculated OR of risk for these diseases in individuals positive for associated HLA-A2 subtype and/or class II. The highest OR was observed in individuals positive for both HLA-A*0206 and –DPB1*0501, or both –A*0207 and –DRB4*0101 in GD or HT, respectively (OR = 7.9 or 6.0 in GD or HT, respectively, Table 3), confirming that both HLA class I and class II are involved in controlling susceptibility to AITD at allele level.

Table 2 Association of HLA-A2 subtypes and AITD

HLA-A allele	% Control (n=553)	% Graves (n=87)	% Hashimoto (n=100)
A*0201	20.0	27.6	23.0
*0206	15.3	32.2 a	16.0
*0207	7.2	13.8	17.0 c
*0210	1.3	1.1	1.0
*2402	60.8	48.3 b	60.0
*3302	15.9	9.2	6.0 d

a: RR=2.63, p<0.0005, b: RR=0.60, p<0.05,
c: RR=2.66, p<0.005, d: RR=0.36, p<0.01

Table 3. High risk for AITD in individuals positive for both associated HLA-A2 allele and HLA class II

A*0206	DRB1*0501	Control[a] (n=268)	Graves[a] (n=78)	OR[b]
-	-	91	9	-
+	-	11	3	2.8
-	+	134	50	3.8
+	+	32	25	7.9

A*0207	DRB4*0101	Control[a] (n=268)	Graves[a] (n=100)	OR[b]
-	-	78	10	-
+	-	12	7	4.6
-	+	165	73	3.5
+	+	13	10	6.0

[a] Individuals who have (+) or do not have (-) the HLA alleles are counted.
[b] ORs were calculated using the group of individuals who were negaive for both A2 and class II as a reference.

Peptide binding motif of HLA-A2 subtypes

Our next question was whether peptide binding motif is different each other in HLA-A2 subtypes. To address this question we eluted and sequenced the naturally processed peptides from three HLA-A2 subtypes (HLA-A*0204, -A*0206, and –A*0207) that differ by a single amino acid residue substitution each with HLA-A*0201 at the floor of the binding groove (15). Allele-specific peptide motifs for each HLA-A2 subtype substantially differed from that of HLA-A*0201 in the dominant anchor residues (Table 4). The

Table 4. Anchors of peptides eluted from HLA-A2 subtypes

Subtype	Anchor [a]	Anchor Site	Amino Acid Change

A*0201	Dominant
	Strong
		1 2 3 4 5 6 7 8 9
		L **V**
		  E L L
		  P V
		     I
			-

A*0204	Dominant
	Strong
		1 2 3 4 5 6 7 8 9
		L **L**
		   E L L
		   P I
			97R→97M

A*0206	Dominant
	Strong
		1 2 3 4 5 6 7 8 9
		V
		  Q I E L V
		  L P L
			9F→9Y

A*0207	Dominant Strong	1 2 3 4 5 6 7 8 9 **L D** **L** P E I	99Y→99C

[a] Criteria for putative anchor residues were fulfilled by showing 1) a > 50 % increase in the absolute amount compared with the previous cycle, and 2) a signal intensity stronger than fivefold over the average signal intensity for other residues in the absolute amount, Residues with a 5- to 10-fold strength are designated as strong anchors, and those with a > 10 fold strength as dominant anchors.

relative signal intensities for 18 self peptides, determined by mass spectrometry, precisely reflected these peptide motifs. Some overlapping peptides were isolated from both HLA-A*0201 and a single HLA-A2 variant, but no peptide was ubiquitously found across all variants. To rationalize the differences in peptide motifs, possible conformations of each allele were computer modeled by energy minimization calculations base on the reported crystal structure of HLA-A*0201 (16-18). According to these models, the differences in peptide motifs could be explained by substituted-residue-driven conformational changes for each HLA/peptide complex. These results demonstrated the fine differences in self peptide repertoires in HLA-A2 subtypes. Although we could not identify candidate antigenic peptides for AITD using information of these binding motifs, these would contribute to the prediction of antigenic peptides that provoke autoimmune T cell response in the thyroid.

Models for pathogenesis of AITD

From the genetical and immunological point of view, we propose models for pathogenesis of AITD. In the case of GD, endogenous (or exogenous) unknown peptides bound to HLA-A*0206 might be recognized by CD8$^+$ T cells (CTL) which destroy thyrocytes, and then peptides from TSHR released from thyrocytes are bound to HLA-DP5 to activate Th2 type of CD4$^+$ T cells which can help production of antibody to TSHR. HLA-DP5-restricted CD4$^+$ T cells may help functional maturation of CD8$^+$ T cells which augment destruction of thyrocytes. In case of HT, similar to GD, CTL against endogenous (or exogenous) unknown peptides bound to HLA-A*0207, which are different from peptides bound to HLA-A*0206, may destroy thyrocytes, and then peptides derived from thyroid peroxidase or thyroglobulin bound to HLA-DR53 activate Th1 type of CD4$^+$ T cells which can help CTL activity. To test this model it is essential to : 1) identify genetic factors except for HLA involved in AITD in Japanese population; 2) identify the self or exogenous peptides recognized by CTL ; 3) clarify the molecular mechanisms of resistance to AITD controlled by HLA. Our recent study using genome-wide linkage analysis to search genetic factors (19) as well as understanding the mechanisms of the association between HLA and diseases enable us to develop a method for prevention and treatment of AITD.

Acknowledgment

We thank A. Kimura, N. Kamikawaji, H. Tamai for technical support and advice.

References

1. Uno H, Sasazuki T, Tamai H, Matsumoto H(1981) Two major genes, linked to HLA and Gm, control susceptibility to Graves' disease. Nature 292:768-770

2. Farid NR, Barnard JM, Marshall WH, Woolfrey I, O'Driscoll RF (1977) Thyroid autoimmune disease in a large Newfoundland family: the influence of HLA. J Clin Endocrinol Metab 45:1165-1172

3. Hawkins BR, Ma JT, Lam KS, Wang CC, Yeung RT (1985) Association of HLA antigens with thyrotoxic Graves' disease and periodic paralysis in Hong Kong Chinese. Clin Endocrinol (Oxf) 23:245-252

4. Todd JA, Acha-Orbea H, Bell JI, Chao N, Fronek Z, Jacob CO, McDermott M, Sinha AA, Timmerman L, Steinman L, McDevitt HO. (1988)A molecular basis for MHC class II--associated autoimmunity. Science. 240:1003-1009.

5. Sasazuki T, Nishimura Y, Muto M, Ohta N (1983) HLA-linked genes controlling immune response and disease susceptibility. Immunol Rev. 70:51-75.

6. Tandon N, Mehra NK, Taneja V, Vaidya MC, Kochupillai N (1990) HLA antigens in Asian Indian patients with Graves' disease. Clin Endocrinol . 33:21-26.

7. Inoue D, Sato K, Enomoto T, Sugawa H, Maeda M, Inoko H, Tsuji K, Mori T, Imura H (1992) Correlation of HLA types and clinical findings in Japanese patients with hyperthyroid Graves' disease: evidence indicating the existence of four subpopulations. Clin Endocrinol. 36:75-82.

8. Farid NR, Thompson C (1986) HLA and autoimmune endocrine disease 1985. Mol Biol Med. 3:85-97.

9. Wang FW, Yu ZQ, Xy JJ, Wang XL, Zhang DQ, Chen JL (1988) HLA and hypertrophic Hashimoto's thyroiditis in Shanghai Chinese. Tissue Antigens. 32:235-236.

10. Sakurami T, Ueno Y, Iwaki Y, Park MS, Terasaki PI, Saji H (1982) HLA-DR specificities among Japanese with several autoimmune diseases. Tissue Antigens. 19:129-133.

11. Naito S, Sasaki H, Arakawa K (1987) Japanese Graves' disease: association with HLA-Bw46. Endocrinol Jpn. 34:685-688.

12.Imanishi T, Akaza T, Kimura A, Tokunaga K, Gojobori T. Allele and haplotype frequencies for HLA and complement loci in various ethnic groups. In Tsuji K, Aizawa M, Sasazuki T (eds) 1992; HLA 1991, vol 1. Oxford, Oxford University Press, 1065

13.Dong RP, Kimura A, Okubo R, Shinagawa H, Tamai H, Nishimura Y, Sasazuki T (1992) HLA-A and DPB1 loci confer susceptibility to Graves' disease. Hum Immunol. 35:165-172.

14.Wan XL, Kimura A, Dong RP, Honda K, Tamai H, Sasazuki T (1995) HLA-A and -DRB4 genes in controlling the susceptibility to Hashimoto's thyroiditis. Hum Immunol. 42:131-136.

15.Zemmour J, Parham P (1993) HLA class I nucleotide sequences, 1992. Immunogenetics. 37:239-250.

16.Bjorkman PJ, Saper MA, Samraoui B, Bennett WS, Strominger JL, Wiley DC (1987) Structure of the human class I histocompatibility antigen, HLA-A2. Nature. 329:506-512.

17.Saper MA, Bjorkman PJ, Wiley DC (1991) Refined structure of the human histocompatibility antigen HLA-A2 at 2.6 A resolution. J Mol Biol. 219:277-319.

18.Madden DR, Garboczi DN, Wiley DC (1993) The antigenic identity of peptide-MHC complexes: a comparison of the conformations of five viral peptides presented by HLA-A2. Cell. 75:693-708.

19.Sakai K, Shirasawa S, Ishikawa N, Ito K, Tamai H, Kuma K, Akamizu T, Tanimura M, Furugaki K, Yamamoto K, Sasazuki T (2001) Identification of susceptibility loci for autoimmune thyroid disease to 5q31-q33 and Hashimoto's thyroiditis to 8q23-q24 by multipoint affected sib-pair linkage analysis in Japanese. Hum Mol Genet. 10:1379-1386.

What Can We Learn from the Genetics of Diabetes?

Donald W. Bowden, Ph.D.
Professor of Biochemistry and Internal Medicine (Endocrinology & Metabolism) Department of Biochemistry Wake Forest University School of Medicine Medical Center Blvd. Winston-Salem, NC 27157, USA
Telephone: 336-716-3912 FAX: 336-716-7200
EMAIL: dbowden@wfubmc.edu

It is a great pleasure to have the opportunity to address you and I thank the organizers and especially Dr. Davies and Dr. Akamizu for inviting me to speak. The topic I was asked to address is: What progress has been made in the search for diabetes genes, and how and what are people looking for in the diabetes area that might contribute to the efforts to identify thyroid disease genes.

Outline

First, I will summarize my thoughts on the question of whether diabetes can really be a model for studies of thyroid disease genetics. Second, I will summarize the status of some of the searches for diabetes genes, and what I believe have been the real major landmarks in that area. Third, what are current trends in diabetes genetics, and what are people doing in diabetes genetics, what are people look for, what is happening technically and organizationally? Finally, I am going talk briefly about positional cloning of candidate diabetes genes using our research on chromosome 20. It is a case study from my own laboratory that, I think, illustrates some of the complexities we face in type 2 diabetes and illustrates where the search for genes involved in thyroid disease might actually have some advantages. Then, at least from my limited perspective, I will summarize what I believe are trends in complex disease genetics.

Key words

diabetes, autoimmune thyroid disease, MODY, HLA, chromosome 2q, chromosome 20, calpain 10, GLUT10, glucose transporter 10

Genes and Disease

We are all interested in genes that contribute to disease: How can we locate them? How can we identify them? In addition, we are facing something in diabetes research that we did not think about a whole lot in the early days: once we find a gene, how do we characterize it and how do we understand how it works, and how can we link that back to the disease?

What kinds of genes might contribute to the diseases in which we are interested? Although my lab has been involved in monogenic disorders and studied monogenic disorders for many years, including medullary thyroid carcinoma, I am going to focus on common disease in the general population. It is widely accepted that most, if not all, common diseases have a genetic component. In contrast to many monogenic disorders, this genetic component contributes genetic susceptibility; but this genetic susceptibility is expressed as a function of the environment in which an individual lives and the lifestyle they lead. Therefore, we are talking about the sum of genes, lifestyle, and environment, as several other contributors have addressed already. The sum of these three issues is what contributes to susceptibility.

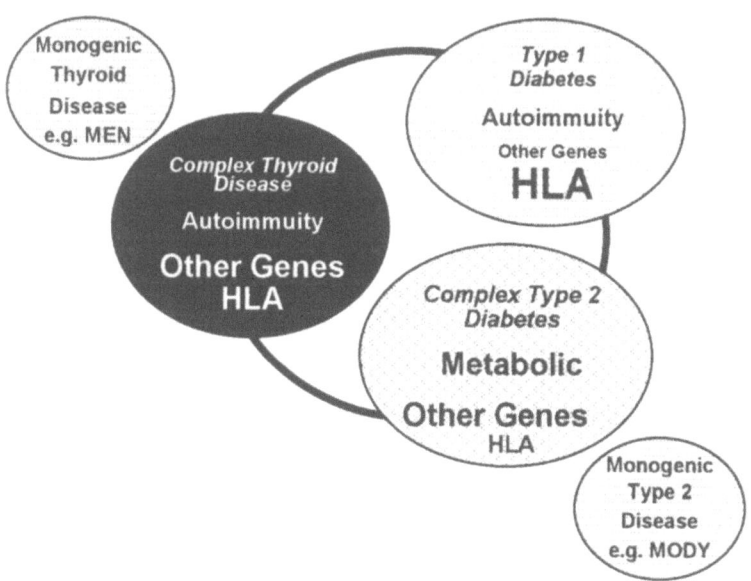

Figure 1. The genetic components of thyroid disease: similarities and differences with diabetes.

Thyroid Genetics from a Diabetologist's Perspective

How does thyroid disease appear from a diabetologist's perspective (Figure 1)? How does thyroid disease fit into the spectrum of diseases? There are two major forms of diabetes: Type I and Type 2. Type I diabetes is characterized by autoimmunity targeted to the pancreatic eyelet cells. The major genetic component of Type I diabetes is the HLA gene region, which contributes much more than any other part of the genome. There are some modifying genes but, relatively speaking, these are rather modest in their impact on risk to develop diabetes compared to HLA.

In contrast, in Type 2 diabetes there has historically been only modest evidence that HLA may contribute to Type 2 diabetes risk, consequently the tiny HLA letters in the Type 2 diabetes circle in Figure 1. Type 2 diabetes is characterized as a metabolic disease. While there are uncommon monogenic forms of Type 2 diabetes (the MODY forms of diabetes) the great majority of the disease seems to be relatively heterogeneous in its clinical expression between individuals and in different populations. A particular puzzle for Type 2 diabetes is that we do not really know what the target organ is, though we know a number of organs that seem to be involved. Many of us would think that Type 2 is more of a systemic rather than targeted disease.

Finally, how do I look at thyroid disease? I think thyroid disease and the autoimmune form of thyroid disease falls somewhere in between the characteristics of Type I and Type 2 diabetes. It is interesting that Dr. Davies spoke earlier that some people say: "Well just let the diabetes people figure it out and then we will follow along." Actually, I do not think that this is a very good suggestion. The fact that all participants at this conference have independently pursued autoimmune thyroid disease is very valid. The most striking difference Type 1 diabetes and, say Graves disease, is that while HLA clearly contributes to susceptibility in autoimmune thyroid disease, there is a dramatic difference in the magnitude of the affect compared to Type 1 diabetes. HLA does not seem to be the major contributor for genetic risk in thyroid disease. Thyroid researchers have the advantage, though, compared to Type 2 diabetes in that a likely suspect in the thyroid disease etiology is autoimmunity and a mechanism of autoimmunity is a major target for autoimmune thyroid disease. Therefore, with thyroid diseases we have an autoimmune disease that is most likely to be dominated by non-HLA genes.

Genetic Studies of Diabetes

Why study diabetes using genetic approaches? A brief look at the complexity of intermediary metabolism suggests that the pathways leading to and from glucose, the hallmark of diabetes are so complex that simply picking which step in which pathway might be defective in diabetes is impossible. Even the simplest view of metabolism reflects the complexities of the disease we are trying to study: the metabolic complexity of Type 2 diabetes. Equally as complex is the regulation of the immune responses that characterize Type I diabetes.

Researches in both Type I and Type 2 diabetes have taken the positional cloning approach in efforts to identify disease genes, just as many other genetic researchers looking at complex diseases. The steps in this approach are a global survey of all the chromosomes (usually in family studies), which, if everything works as we hope, will identify certain parts of certain chromosomes as candidate regions for containing susceptibility genes. This initial phase is followed by a screening of candidate genes in those regions and then hopefully, eventually, identification and characterization of mutations.

Diabetes researchers have been drawn to genetic methods due to frustration with conventional approaches to try to identify diabetes genes and the origins of diabetes. Additional frustration comes from the fact that, in contrast to thyroid disease, clinical treatments available for diabetes are largely unsatisfactory in their ability to prevent long-term complications of diabetes. For these reasons, very early on diabetes researchers have been in the forefront of the application of genetic technologies to studying complex disease. Among the important studies are originally the HLA association and linkage with Type I diabetes, which actually goes back many many years. Second, linkage studies of Maturity Onset Diabetes of the Young (MODY) have led to the identification of several genes causing monogenic forms of diabetes. These studies have been of special interest since they have proven one hypothesis of genetic studies: that they have the capacity to identify novel pathways leading, in this case, to the realization that mutations in simple transcription factors, can lead to diabetes. Probably the first genome scan for complex disease was carried out in Type I diabetes by John Todd's group (Davies et al. 1994). And now, most recently, what is potentially the first positional cloning of a complex disease gene, the calpain 10 gene identification in Mexican American Type 2 diabetes families (Horikawa et al., 2000).

One of the landmark papers in complex disease and diabetes research was John Todd's genome scan searching for human Type I diabetes susceptibility genes that was first published in 1994 (Davis et al., 1994). In this first genome scan they searched for Type I diabetes genes in 280 families with multiple Type I affected children and detected evidence for linkage on a number of chromosomes. Key features of the genome scan were the use of automated equipment to genotype microsatellite polymorphisms in the Type I diabetes families. They found several chromosomal locations that they suggested were locations for linkage to Type I diabetes. One important conclusion that can be drawn from the paper was that the HLA region is by far the major susceptibility locus for Type I diabetes. This result really contrasts with the results that have been seen in similar studies now performed in autoimmune thyroid disease. An expression of how important HLA is was the observation that the HLA LOD score was 19.3, and the next closest autosomal non-HLA linkage was a very modest LOD score of 1.6.

The most dramatic, perhaps the most exciting and, in many ways, maybe the most perplexing development in Type 2 diabetes research is the publication just this month of another landmark paper (Horikawa et al., 2000): the description of the association of the calpain10 gene, a calcium activated protease with Type 2 diabetes in Mexican Americans. This was the first identification by positional cloning of a gene that contributes to a common complex disease.

The paper by Horikawa and colleagues, including Graeme Bell, Nancy Cox, and many others, is the summary of a long ongoing study that, using a genome screen, originally suggested the presence of a Mexican American Type 2 diabetes gene on chromosome 2q. In 1999, they demonstrated that there is apparently an interaction between genes on chromosome 2 and chromosome 15 (Cox et al., 1999). Now, in the Horikawa et al. paper they have sequenced 66 kilobases in an interval containing three genes. They have identified 179 SNP polymorphisms or single nucleotide polymorphisms in that region and they have demonstrated that a combination of three SNPs in that region is associated with Mexican American Type 2 diabetes. What makes the observations difficult to put into context is the fact that these 3 SNPs are in the non-coding regions of the calpain 10 gene: a calcium activated protease. This actually creates more questions than are answered in this paper. Is this really the gene? There are two alternatives here. One possibility is that using sophisticated genetic methodology they have revealed hitherto unknown mechanism for the development of diabetes. A second alternative is they are wrong: calpain 10 is not the origin of the disease. At this time, we do not know what the true answer is. So is it a new insight into the origins of Type 2 diabetes? The one thing that is really overpowering, is the research effort and commitment of resources that was needed to carry out this study. This is the result of an extraordinary effort: they sequenced 66 kilobases in twenty different people. So they generated over a million base pairs of data and then evaluated a vast number of SNPs, 179, in a huge number of patients. At the end of that enormous expenditure of resources we still do not really known what is going on.

What is the future direction of diabetes genetics?

What is in store for the future? What kinds of tools are available for Type 2 diabetes research that may also be relevant for autoimmune thyroid disease? The complete sequence of the human genome is on the verge of being completed. The draft sequence now is useful in some places, but it is not very useful at all in other chromosomal locations. The interface between user and data especially will need to be improved in the near future to make the sequence a more useful tool. High density SNP maps of validated single nucleotide type polymorphisms are going to greatly accelerate our ability to do association studies and may also be useful for highly automated genome screens (with some caveats about their analytical utility). Another important source of data for the researcher that will come in the future are expression profiles of all of the human genes. Consequently, if a researcher can rapidly identify a set of genes in a region linked to a phenotype in genetic studies, expression profiles may be very valuable in identifying candidates for further analysis. Finally, a very important source of information for researchers interested in human disease is a catalog DNA sequence diversity: a compendium of sequence differences. This is being created gradually now as part of the SNP consortium and is clearly an important next phase of the Genome Project.

There are two major developments in diabetes research that are relevant to thyroid genetic studies: first are the increasing collaborative efforts between different groups as we realize the complexity of the diabetes problem is much bigger than we originally envisioned. Second, an increasingly sophisticated clinical analysis of patients in our studies. Such a sophisticated clinical analysis is shown in Figure 2. This is actually just one example from my laboratory where we are also interested in cardiovascular diseases associated with Type 2 diabetes. Here we have CT scans of the hearts from three sisters, two that are diabetic and one of who is not diabetic. The use of sophisticated technology can provide us with some genuine insights into what is going on in the disease. In Figure 2 we are looking at the coronary calcification of coronary arteries using CT scans. So, a sophisticated and expensive methodology, but in this case, we can non-invasively image the coronary arteries of people who, in this case, two people with very large amounts of calcium who have Type 2 diabetes compared to their sister who does not have diabetes and has a very modest amount of calcium.

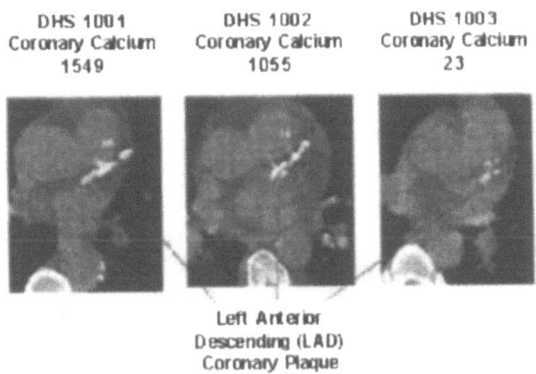

DHS 1001
Coronary Calcium
1549

DHS 1002
Coronary Calcium
1055

DHS 1003
Coronary Calcium
23

Left Anterior
Descending (LAD)
Coronary Plaque

Figure 2. CT Scans of coronary arteries of three sisters, two with Type 2 diabetes (DHS 1001 and DHS 1002) and a third non-diabetic sister (DHS 1003)

The other emerging trend in diabetes genetics is more collaboration between different research groups. For example, the last several years has seen the organization of an international consortium to pool Type 2 diabetes linkage data (International Type 2 Diabetes Linkage Analysis Consortium) and there is an emerging consortium or developing consortium to do the same thing with Type I diabetes data. The International Type 2 Diabetes Linkage Analysis Consortium has over 15 different laboratories contributing data from all over the world. This has facilitated the collection of an enormous amount of data from many different areas. The total number of families with multiple Type 2 diabetes affected individuals in them approaches 3000. The total number of genotyped individuals is 18,900: an enormous number. The total number of affected individuals is over 8,000. With these large numbers comes considerable statistical power to detect linked regions in family studies.

The initial focus for the linkage analysis consortium was on human chromosome 20. A number of research groups, including my own, previously developed data or evidence that there was linkage to Type 2 diabetes on chromosome 20. With the pooling of data from many groups, the evidence for the existence of a Type 2 diabetes gene on chromosome 20 remains strong.

The Search for Type 2 Diabetes Genes on Chromosome 20

The data supporting evidence for Type 2 diabetes susceptibility genes on chromosome-20 has motivated a number of groups to search for the diabetogenic genes using the conventional positional cloning approach. The first step has been to try to locate genes by global linkage analysis studies in families followed by trying to narrow the location by local or association studies.

The one striking think about chromosome 20 and Type 2 diabetes is the evidence from multiple laboratories suggesting the existence of Type 2 diabetes genes on 20. The focus of my laboratory on 20 derives from these observations in multiple studies of Caucasian Type 2 diabetes families. These include two studies from the United States: one from my laboratory (Bowden et al., 1997) and one from Andrzej Krolewski's laboratory at the Joslin Diabetes Center in Boston (Ji et al., 1997). Then a study of French Type 2 diabetes families from Phillippe Froguel's group in France (Zouali et al., 1997). Finally, studies of Finnish Type 2 diabetes families in the Fusion study (Ghosh et al., 1999). Consistent with results of searches for complex disease genes, the results of any individual study are not very compelling evidence of linkage. Combined, however, there is a strong suggestion that something important is going on. When you put data from multiple groups together, there is consistent evidence of linkage around in the same region. In an aside relevant to some of the discussions of searches for thyroid disease genes, what we find when we put all our data together is that there are multiple overlapping peaks that are not at the same position. What we find are peaks in this area of the long arm of chromosome 20.

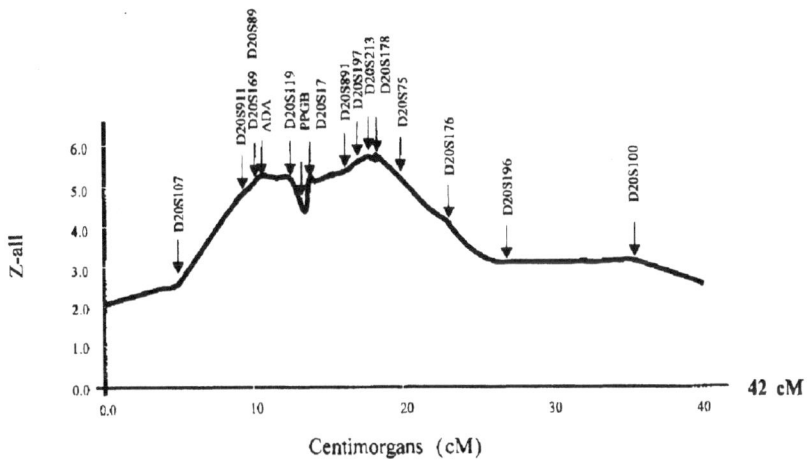

Figure 3. Multipoint linkage analysis of genetic markers in 20q12-q13.1 in Type 2 diabetes families. Z-all, the lod score is measured on the Y-axis and location along the chromosome (in centimorgans from the origin) is shown on the X-axis.

Figure 3 shows the result of linkage analysis on chromosome 20 in our Type 2 families merged with the data from Andrzej Krolewski's families from Boston. This figure shows a non-parametric lod score calculated on the left with the lod score being graphed as a function of position on chromosome 20. A peak with a bimodal shape with a relatively good magnitude, over 5 here, is observed. We followed up that particular study doing linkage analysis with an association analysis. In this case, we looked at microsatellite markers all along this region of chromosome 20, along 20q12 through 13.1 (Figure 4). As with the linkage data, we observed two apparent association peaks. One association peak is at the location for the adenosine deaminase gene (ADA) and another at the location for a microsatellite marker D20S888. Interestingly enough, these two peaks, though it may just be coincidental, are more or less right under the seemingly bimodal linkage analysis peak (Figure 3). We are not totally convinced that this is exactly what is going on, but at least the two results are consistent.

These genetic studies presented us with two regions to investigate in detail leading to the physical mapping of these regions. Consequently, we have been trying to define the gene containing region and cloning chromosomal fragments. What was a major effort in the past is now becoming much easier with the continuing development of the DNA sequence database from the Human Genome Project and this phase of analysis may not even be needed at all in the future. The first step in this phase in this step of positional cloning was to generate a detailed physical map of the region initially using YAC and BAC clones to cover the 10 Mb region. We have now extended that to a detailed expressed sequence map of the region that involves identifying genes in the region and evaluating their potential involvement in diabetes.

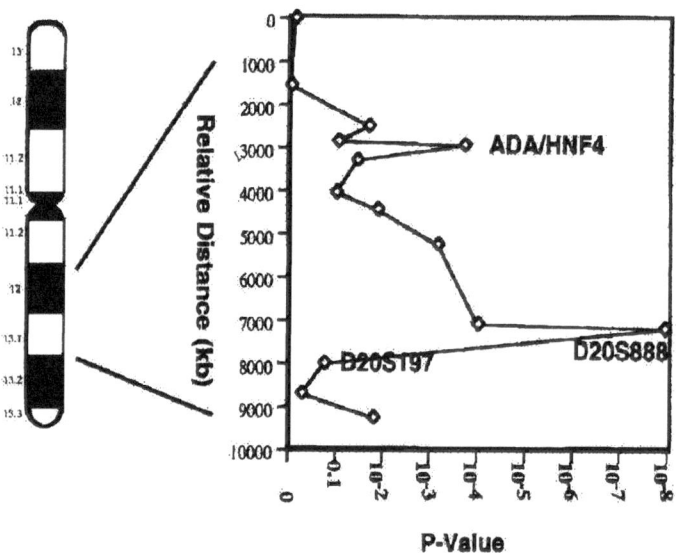

Figure 4. Association analysis on chromosome 20q12-q13.1

We have looked at quite a few genes in the 20q12-q13.1 region and that actually presents a significant problem in Type 2 diabetes. The beauty of autoimmune thyroid disease is one can at least project that a disease gene is highly likely to have an autoimmune component to it. For Type 2 diabetes, we really do not know where to look. It could be involved in the insulin signaling pathway, it could be metabolic, could even be a transcription factors. That is because mutations in transcription factors can cause MODY. We have looked at many genes, evaluating them for different alleles (different sequences), and then trying to find out whether there was any evidence for association with diabetes. While doing these experiments, one particular gene caught our eye. In the human genome sequence data, it was designated as a membrane transporter-like protein and was very near the genetic marker D20S888 that was associated with diabetes in our earlier genetic studies.

When we took the sequence of the membrane transporter like gene and BLASTed it against the GenBank sequence database we observed that it was primarily similar to genes that were sugar transporters. This was of interest to us since if this gene is a glucose transporter it could well be a good candidate for a diabetes gene. Impaired glucose transport has been implicated in decreased insulin stimulated muscle glycogen synthesis and in insulin resistance, two hallmarks of diabetes (Cline et al., 1999; Shepherd et al., 1999). With this interesting observation, we began to analyze this gene in detail. We cloned a cDNA from a placental cDNA library and found a five exon gene which has 1,623 base pairs of coding sequence, encompasses 26.8 kilobases of genomic DNA and that encodes for a 541 amino acid protein. This gene has been designated GLUT10 (glucose transporter 10).

When the sequence of GLUT10, our novel gene, is compared with other known glucose transporters using multiple sequence alignment, GLUT10 shares between 23 and 32% amino acid identity with glucose transporters 1-5. An analysis of the amino acid sequence of GLUT10 predicts a protein with 12 transmembrane domains similar to other glucose transporters. In addition, GLUT10 shares a number of sequence characteristics with other glucose transporters. Based on the sequence characteristics we were fairly well convinced that it is a glucose transporter. Figure 5 shows the results of a phylogenetic analysis of the family of glucose transporters. GLUT10 is furthest from the GLUT1 glucose transporter and closest to the recently identified GLUT8 transporter, which was just published this year (Doege et al., 2000).

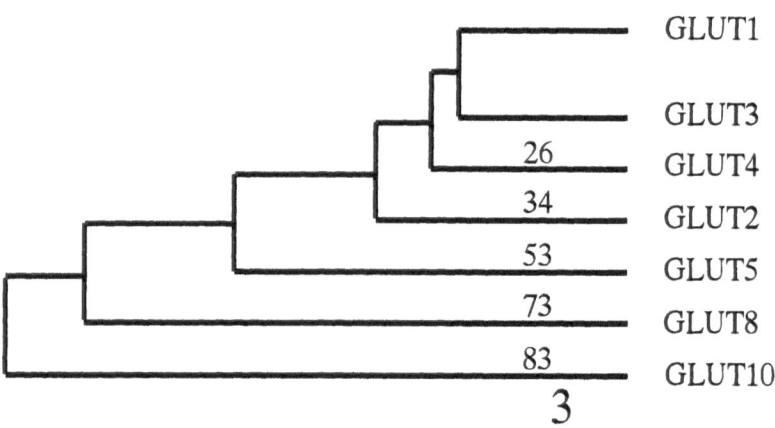

Figure 5. Phylogram of glucose transporters including GLUT10. The distances between glucose transporters are annotated as amino acid changes for 100 amino acids

By Northern Blot analysis of different tissues GLUT10 is expressed in tissues that we might expect for a gene that could be involved in diabetes. Among these are liver, skeletal muscle, and pancreas, in addition to heart and lung. By RT-PCR analysis, a number of other tissues show evidence of GLUT10 expression. It might be of interest to you that the thyroid and adrenal glands also show expression in the RT-PCR analysis.

In order to test whether this new gene was indeed a glucose transporter, we injected Xenopus oocytes with mRNA for GLUT10 and performed glucose uptake assays using the non-metabolizable substrate 2-deoxy-D-glucose. Figure 6 shows the results of this analysis. We compared the glucose transport activity of GLUT10 to several other known glucose transporters: GLUT3 and GLUT4. As can be seen in Figure 6, GLUT10 transports glucose at a rate that is similar to the activity of known glucose transporters GLUT3 and GLUT4. We also looked at the specificity of that transport by competition experiments in which 2-deoxy-D-glucose transport was competed with other potential substrates such as galactose, deoxyglucose, and D-glucose. In the competition experiments, D-glucose competes better than galactose, but the non-metabolizable substrate 2-deoxy-D-glucose almost completely eliminates transport. In addition, phloretin, an inhibitor of transporters, also reduces the transport of glucose. Consequently, we have fairly strong evidence now that GLUT10 is indeed a glucose transporter.

The relatively low activity of GLUT10 was reminiscent to us of the glucose transporter 4 (GLUT4). GLUT4 shows significantly increased transport activity in the presence of insulin. That is, it is an insulin responsive glucose transporter. We carried out such an experiment comparing the insulin stimulation of GLUT4 and GLUT10 and we found that both GLUT4 and GLUT10 activity is insulin stimulated in the oocyte uptake assay.

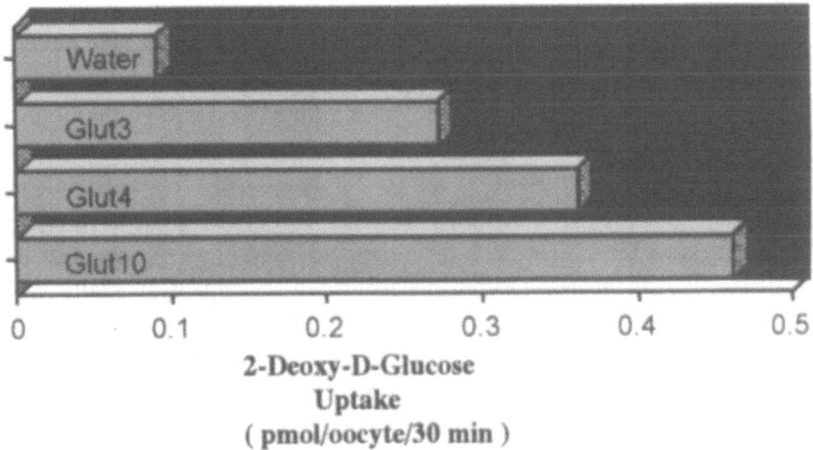

Figure 6. 2-deoxy-D-glucose uptake assays in mRNA injected oocytes.

Summary of Chromosome 20 Studies

In summary, there is evidence that one or more diabetes genes are located on human chromosome 20. We have carried out an exhaustive analysis of this region of the human genome and have evaluated several candidate diabetes genes in this region. In particular we have carried out a detailed sequence analysis and functional analysis of one gene, GLUT10, which appears to be a novel glucose transporter. It is located in the q12-q13.1 on chromosome 20, a region previously linked to Type 2 diabetes. So the location and function of GLUT10 and its insulin responsiveness makes an attractive candidate diabetes gene. We are involved now in trying to find out if certain alleles that we have identified in GLUT10 are associated with diabetes and have functional differences with the common form of the gene.

Overview and the Future

There are many barriers to identifying genes that contribute to complex diseases such as Type 2 diabetes or autoimmune thyroid disease. The hurdles are tremendous and I have tried to touch on them with this glucose transporter 10 story. The functional analysis of the role that a novel gene may play in disease susceptibility can be very laborious and time consuming. If it is not a gene that is well characterized, trying to figure out how it works may be very difficult. Even with a complete sequence of genes in the model system yeast, only about 50% of the genes have any information on their functional role. That means a great deal of effort is going to have to go into understanding how genes of unknown function work. Understanding the genetic origin of human diseases will still require a lot of careful clinical evaluation and identifying the origins of complex diseases may be even more complex than previously imagined. That could be the most important lesson from the calpain 10 story. Are the polymorphisms identified in calpain 10 really contributing to diabetes, and in what way are they contributing to diabetes? Most of us have evaluated only exons and promoters of genes in our search for disease alleles. In the future, it will probably be necessary to look comprehensively at the entire genomic sequence containing a gene. This means that enormous amounts of DNA sequencing will be necessary and this will be very intensive and very expensive. One of the clearest lessons from diabetes research is that genetic studies of complex disease are getting bigger and more complex. The methodology and technology is becoming more sophisticated and it is definitely becoming more expensive. The problem of finding complex disease genes is harder than was envisioned five or ten years ago, but there is substantial reason for optimism for the future.

Acknowledgements

This work was supported by grants from the National Institutes of Health (USA) R01 DK41269, R01DK56289, R01 DK53591, and a grant from the American Diabetes Association, and is the result of contributions from numerous collaborators and thousands of patient participants.

References

1. Bowden DW. Sale M. Howard TD. Qadri A (1997) Spray BJ. Rothschild CB. Akots G. Rich SS. Freedman BI. Linkage of genetic markers on human chromosomes 20 and 12 to NIDDM in Caucasian sib pairs with a history of diabetic nephropathy. Diabetes. 46(5):882-6

2. Cline GW. Petersen KF. Krssak M. Shen J. Hundal RS. Trajanoski Z. Inzucchi S. Dresner A. Rothman DL. Shulman GI (1999) Impaired glucose transport as a cause of decreased insulin-stimulated muscle glycogen synthesis in type 2 diabetes. New England Journal of Medicine. 341(4):240-6

3. Cox NJ. Frigge M. Nicolae DL. Concannon P. Hanis CL. Bell GI. Kong A (1999) Loci on chromosomes 2 (NIDDM1) and15 interact to increase susceptibility to diabetes in Mexican Americans. Nature Genetics. 21(2):213-5

4. Davies JL. Kawaguchi Y. Bennett ST. Copeman JB (1994) Cordell HJ. Pritchard LE. Reed PW. Gough SC. Jenkins SC. Palmer SM. et al. A genome-wide search for human type 1 diabetes susceptibility genes [see comments]. [Journal Article Nature. 371(6493):130-6

5. Doege H. Schurmann A. Bahrenberg G. Brauers A. Joost HG (2000) GLUT8, a novel member of the sugar transport facilitator family with glucose transport activity. Journal of Biological Chemistry. 275(21):16275-80

6. Ghosh S. Watanabe RM. Hauser ER. Valle T. Magnuson VL. Erdos MR. Langefeld CD. Balow J Jr. Ally DS. Kohtamaki K. Chines P. Birznieks G. Kaleta HS. Musick A. Te C. Tannenbaum J. Eldridge W. Shapiro S. Martin C. Witt A. So A. Chang J. Shurtleff B. Porter R. Boehnke M. et al. (1999) Type 2 diabetes: evidence for linkage on chromosome 20 in 716 Finnish affected sib pairs. Proceedings of the National Academy of Sciences of the United States of America. 96(5):2198-203

7. Horikawa Y, Oda N, Cox NJ, Li X, Orho-Melander M, Hara M, et al. (2000) Genetic variation in the gene encoding calpain-10 is associated with type 2 diabetes mellitus. Nature Genetics Volume 26 Number 2: 163-175

8. Ji L. Malecki M. Warram JH. Yang Y. Rich SS. Krolewski AS (1997) New susceptibility locus for NIDDM is localized to human chromosome 20q. Diabetes. 46(5):876-81

9. Shepherd PR. Kahn BB. (1999) Glucose transporters and insulin action--implications for insulin resistance and diabetes mellitus. New England Journal of Medicine. 341(4):248-57

10. Zouali H. Hani EH. Philippi A. Vionnet N. Beckmann JS. Demenais F. Froguel P (1997) A susceptibility locus for early-onset non-insulin dependent (type 2) diabetes mellitus maps to chromosome 20q, proximal to the phosphoenolpyruvate carboxykinase gene. Human Molecular Genetics. 6(9):1401-8

The Genomic Biology of the Human Chromosome 2q33 Costimulatory Receptor Region

Vincent Ling[1] and Gregory J. Fisk
Genetics Institute/Wyeth Research
87 Cambridge Park Drive Cambridge MA 02140, USA
phone: 617-665-5539 fax: 617-665-5584
E-mail: VLing@genetics.com
[1]To whom correspondence should be addressed.

Abstract

The CTLA4 receptor gene locus on human chromosome 2q33 has been linked to numerous autoimmune diseases including IDDM and AITD. To determine the identity of genes other than CTLA4 that may contribute to immune disease function, 2q33 BAC clones flanking the CTLA4 gene were sequenced. Assembly of 381,403 bp of sequence from three BAC clones and other genomic data revealed a contiguous costimulatory receptor cluster in the order of CD28, CTLA4 and ICOS with a HERV-H type endogenous retrovirus 366 bp downstream of ICOS in reverse orientation. Genomic DNA based microarray expression analysis of subcloned CTLA4/ICOS BAC DNA using PMA-ionomycin activated T-cell versus non-activated T-cell RNA revealed differential hybridization associated with sequences encoding CTLA4, ICOS and endogenous retrovirus (HERV-H). Further examination by Northern blot analysis revealed antisense ICOS transcripts by HERV-H LTRs suggesting a possible mechanism for ICOS gene regulation. Four non-linked polymorphic simple repetitive sequence elements were identified in this region in addition to the known polymorphic CTLA4 3' microsatellite repeat, adding to the repertoire of markers available to assess 2q33 association with autoimmune diseases.

Key words

CTLA4, IDDM, chromosome 2q33, ICOS, endogenous retrovirus, HERV-H, autoimmune thyroid diseases, Graves disease, Hashimoto's disease, CD28, B7-1, B7-2, costimulation, costimulator, costimulatory

Introduction

Human chromosome 2q33 has been extensively studied as a locus associated with autoimmune diseases including autoimmune thyroid diseases (Graves disease and Hashimoto's disease), Addison's disease, insulin-dependent diabetes mellitus (IDDM), myasthenia with thymoma, multiple sclerosis, rheumatoid arthritis, and celiac disease (Kristiansen et al., 2000). Detailed investigation of some of these genetic associations are described elsewhere in this volume. Of the genes residing in 2q33, CTLA4 has been implicated as a critical immune response gene. Potential polymorphisms in a microsatellite repeat located in the 3'-UTR has been tenuously implicated as the contributing to autoimmunity, although no study has yet convincingly demonstrated this phenomena in a controlled experimental setting. Despite the positional evidence of autoimmune disease association to CTLA4 on 2q33, other diseases have also been associated to 2q33 including familial primary pulmonary hypertension (PPH) which as a clinical entity, has with some association with autoimmunity, but now appears to be closely linked to mutations in the bone morphogenetic receptor - II gene (Deng et al., 2000a). Multiple disease linkages to 2q33 suggest that this area of chromosome 2 may be a rich region of potentially important, immunologically related genes. Given that some immune-related genes cluster together on the chromosome, we sought to determine the primary sequence of the 2q33 costimulatory receptor locus with the purpose of better delineating genetic association with the physical location of target genes in this region.

Immunological activation of T-cells is accomplished by a two-signal mechanism utilizing protein ligand and receptor pairs. Signal one results from recognition of antigenic peptide-MHC complexes by the antigen-specific T cell receptor. The second costimulatory signal is delivered by B7-1 / B7-2 ligands located on the antigen presenting cell to the CD28 or CTLA4 receptor located on the T-cell (Abbas and Sharpe, 1999). Signaling through CD28 results in protein phosphorylation and cell proliferative responses (Ward, 1996). The initial reports of CTLA4 as being a second costimulatory receptor were due to the observations that both soluble CD28 and soluble CTLA4 antibodies cause mitogenic responses in T-cell assays. However the preponderance of current evidence suggests that CTLA4 is a negative signaling receptor where engagement to B7-1 or B7-2 ligands results in the down-modulation of T cell activation. It was later understood that although soluble CD28 antibodies delivered a true agonistic costimulatory signal, soluble CTLA4 antibodies were antagonistic and thus blocked naturally occurring negative signaling pathway. Thus the blockade of negative signaling would appeared as a positive signal. A number of conflicting reports have been published debating whether CTLA4 signal transduction pathways involves protein phosphorylation. As of yet no clear-cut, unified mechanism has yet to emerge from the synthesis of the disparate data (Sansom, 2000) that adequately explains the mechanism of CTLA4 action.

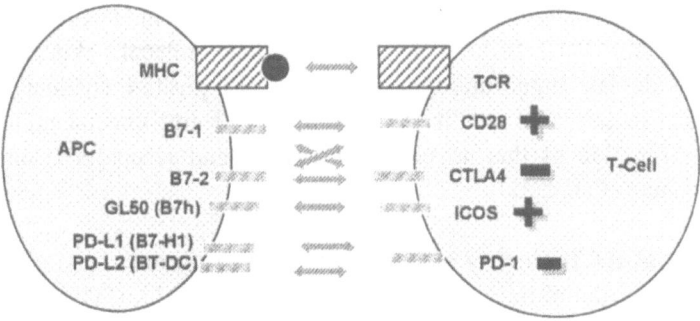

Figure 1. Diagram of current interactions between costimulatory ligands and receptors.

Recently, a CD28-like receptor ICOS (Hutloff et al., 1999) was identified in both mouse and humans systems. CD28 and ICOS exhibit protein sequence identity of ~24 %. Despite structural similarity, ICOS receptor is unlikely to utilize the B7:CD28/CTLA4 costimulatory pathways because of the inability of ICOS-ligand to bind CD28/CTLA4 proteins and of the inability of B7 proteins to bind ICOS receptors (Ling et al., 1999). In vitro analysis of ICOS mediated T-cell costimulation revealed that ICOS engagement resulted in enhanced T cell proliferation and Th-2 cytokine production. Blockade of the ICOS pathway by addition of ICOS-Ig to MLR (mixed lymphocyte reaction) or tetanus toxoid recall response assays resulted in decreased T-cell proliferation (Aicher et al., 2000). Transgenic mice expressing ICOS-ligand exhibited an increase in B-cell germinal center size and enhancement of immunoglobin production (Yoshinaga et al., 1999) suggesting that overexpression of the ligand may influence B cell development. Recently, three independent efforts generated ICOS deficient mice, each group reporting consistent phenotypic findings: ICOS deficiency led to upregulation of gamma IFN, defect in immunoglobulin class switching, impaired germinal center formation, and increased susceptibility to EAE. Taken together, these data are consistent with the model of the ICOS receptor serving as a pivotal signaling molecule involved with secondary T-cell and B-cell proliferation and differentiation. Very recently, a novel set of second signal interaction pairs have been described consisting of the B7-like molecules PD-L1 and PD-L2 ligands with PD-1 receptor, a CTLA-4 like molecule. Like the initial studies of CTLA4 activity, current contradictory reports exist concerning mode of PD-1 signaling; some claim PD-1 to be a negative signaling molecule akin to CTLA4, others provide data suggesting this receptor to be a positive costimulator. Future studies in this area are likely to lead to a clearer understanding of the molecular function of this novel set of ligands and receptors (Dong et al., 2000; Freeman et al., 2000)

Chromosomal Clustering of Immune-related Genes

Despite the distinct functional properties of CD28, CTLA4, ICOS and PD-1 during costimulation, these four receptors are related in sequence structure, with all four belonging to the Ig-superfamily of proteins. All four receptors share a single IgV-like extracellular domain, a transmembrane region and a cytoplasmic domain with intracellular signaling motifs (ITIMs and ITAMs). Similarity in structure also was reflected in the chromosomal localization of CD28 and CTLA4. During the early studies of CTLA4 and CD28 genes, both receptors were found to co-localize to one ~150 kb YAC clone (Balzano et al., 1992). The phenomena of immunological gene clustering has been demonstrated with the initial mapping of 5q31 followed by non-contiguous sequencing of a 680 kb region revealing the presence of IL-3, IL-4, IL-5, IL-13, and GM-CSF genetic loci (Frazer et al., 1997). Remarkably, these cytokine genes do not share remarkable similarity at the nucleotide or protein sequence level, but have been demonstrated to share some overlap in tertiary structure and biological activities. In addition, the sequence determination of chromosome 21 revealed an immunological gene cluster containing the type

II cytokine receptor genes including IFNAR2, IL10R2, IFNAR1 and IFNGR2 (Hattori et al., 2000). It has previously been determined that human PD-1 was located on chromosome 2q37 (Finger et al., 1997) and thus not closely linked to CTLA4. The degree of structural similarity found between the ICOS receptor and CD28 combined with the genetic proximity of CD28 to CTLA4 led us to examine whether the ICOS receptor gene was also clustered with to the 2q33 region of the human genome (Ling et al., in press).

Genomic Sequencing of 2q33 related BAC clones

To determine the distance between the CTLA4, CD28, and ICOS genes, 6 independent BAC clones were isolated by hybridization to costimulatory receptor cDNA probes. Of the BAC clones, two exhibited hybridization with CD28, two with CTLA4, one with ICOS, and one with both CTLA4 and ICOS. Physical mapping of the BAC clones resulted in a hypothetical map of the costimulatory receptor region clustered in the order of CD28, CTLA4, and ICOS (Figure 1). Three-fold shotgun sequencing of BAC 22700 library resulted in 70 contigs spanning approximately 170 kb, while two-fold sequencing of BAC 22606 and BAC 22608 libraries generated 107 contigs spanning 130 kb, and 111 contigs spanning 107 kb, respectively. In addition, mouse BAC 23114 containing CTLA4 and ICOS genes was sequenced two-fold resulting into 143 contigs spanning 131 kb. Gap closure was performed by direct sequencing of BAC clone DNA using primers designed from the sequences flanking contig gaps. When necessary, overlaps to publicly available genomic data were used to position contigs, especially PAC clone p61e2 (Accession #AF225900) bridging the 52,408 bp gap between BAC clone 22606 to BAC clone 22700. Merging sequence data resulted in one finished contiguous sequence of 381,403 bp initiating 42,570 bp upstream of CD28, and ending 85,985 bp downstream of ICOS (Figure 2).

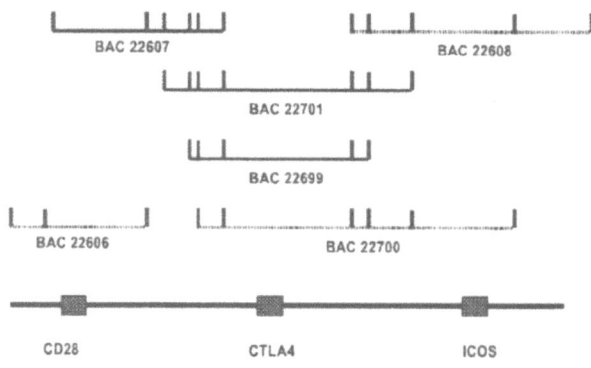

Figure 2. Physical mapping of the costimulatory receptor region. BAC clones 22606, 22700, and 22608 were subse quently sequenced.

Annotation of the Human 2q33 Costimulatory Receptor Gene Cluster

The 381 kb of assembled genomic sequence from the human chromosome 2q33 immunological costimulatory receptor region was further annotated. Twenty potential protein coding elements were identified within the 381 kb costimulatory receptor region with sequences exhibiting either identity to or homology with known DNA: NADH:ubiquinone oxidoreductase homolog, CD28 (NM_006139), keratin-18 pseudogene, nucleophosmin pseudogene, CTLA4, Unigene HS.30542 homolog, ESTs, ICOS, and an element similar to many human endogenous retrovirus type H (RTLV-H or HERV-H). CD28, CTLA4 and ICOS receptors are closely situated, with 252 kb separating the initiation codon of CD28 and the termination codon of ICOS receptor. The mouse syntenic genomic region shares similar organization with areas of high sequence similarity in certain areas outside the coding region. Within the assembled human 2q33 costimulatory receptor region, 2.5% (9,604 bp) was comprised of low complexity repeats, while 15% was comprised of high complexity repeats leaving ~ 82% DNA available to potentially encode transcriptionally active DNA. Two common pseudogenes were found corresponding to keratin-18, an intermediate filament protein associated with carcinomas (Oshima et al., 1996), and nucleophosmin, a ribosomal assembly protein (Philpott et al., 2000). Although we have not assessed whether these pseudogenes are transcribed or whether they may have biological significance, the potential of these pseudogenes to produce functional proteins is low. Both pseudogenes contain initiation codons but have interspersed multiple non-intronic termination codons in all three reading frames. Another potential psuedogene was identified with high sequence similarity to NADH:ubiquinone /oxidoreductase MLRQ, an 81 amino acid protein that functions in the complex I of the mitochondrial respiratory chain, catalyzing the reaction: NADH + ubiquinone = NAD + ubiquinol(Kim et al., 1997). It is not known whether the NADH:ubiquinone oxidoreductase form presented here (79% identity to MLRQ form) is transcribed and represents a novel member of this protein family. It is interesting to note that all three costimulatory receptors share similar transcriptional orientation, while in contrast the pseudogenes, NADH:ubiquinone oxidoreductase and HERV-H element are all positioned in opposite orientation. The shared directionality of the costimulatory receptors is analogous to the unidirectional pattern revealed for the type II cytokine receptor cluster in the recently sequenced chromosome 21 (Hattori et al., 2000). It has been hypothesized that common orientation between structurally related proteins within the genome may reflect the outcome of initial gene duplication events.

Thirteen EST or EST homologs were identified by Blast search that lay outside known exonic and repetitive sequences (Table 1). Further analysis revealed that most of these ESTs were also found in genomic DNA across different chromosomes, but not associated with any known protein. These results suggest that these transcripts may not actually reflect transcribed gene products, but rather, transcribed genomic DNA driven from cryptic promoter sites, such as LTR-type sequences within complex repetitive elements.

Table 1. ESTs within 2q33 costimulatory receptor region

Gene/EST	Position Start	Position End		Reference
	Start	End	Size	Accession #
EST	74209	74682	473	AA311148
EST	75932	76379	447	N20227
EST	88605	88873	268	AA663852
EST	93458	93983	525	AA744591
EST	94424	94744	320	H89084
EST	95762	96257	495	AW237774
EST	98855	99173	318	L44301
EST homolog	230519	232134	1615	R91770, AW474005, AI434725
EST homolog	241762	242097	335	AW238656, AL037926, AI905493
EST homolog	253467	253534	67	N73819, AI801031, AW079941
EST homolog	257288	257506	218	Unigene cluster homolog HS.30542
EST	260890	261082	192	AA663871
EST homolog	267282	269005	1723	AA558770, AA054182, T90825

Based on a recent mapping study of 2q31-33 with genetic markers, the three receptor loci within this assembled region are situated on chromosome 2 with CD28 being the most centromeric and markers now known to be near ICOS being the most telomeric (Deng et al., 2000b). In addition, 22 STS were identified upon BLAST search of this compiled region of 2q33, of which 4 correlated to endogenous retroviral sequence. Endogenous retroviral elements are abundant in the genome with the HERV-H elements found in ~1000 copies in the genome. It remains to be determined if these 4 STS are specific for the element described here. The commonly used genetic markers for 2q33, D2S307 (SARA 43), D2S72, D2S105, and 19E07-1 were contained within the sequence presented here.

Human and mouse CD28 and CTLA4 share a 4 exon structure (Ling et al., 2000), despite the confusing literature that abounds in this field describing CTLA4 as being comprised of 3 exons plus extra leader sequence (Kristiansen et al., 2000). In contrast both mouse and human ICOS sequence data revealed the organization of the ICOS locus to be comprised of 5 exons. ICOS exon 5 encoded the smallest coding sequence, represented by only 4 amino acids followed by a stop codon. In other respects, exons 1-4 parallel the genomic organization of CTLA4 and CD28 with exon 1 encoding the leader sequence, exon 2 encoding the extracellular Ig-V like domain, exon 3 encoding the transmembrane domain and exon 4 and 5 encoding the cytoplasmic domain.

All three costimulatory receptors shared similar pattern of intron size distribution in which intron 1> intron 3> intron 2.

Ab initio predictions of exons within the costimulatory receptor region of 2q33

The 381 Kb costimulatory receptor locus was analyzed by the exon prediction programs DiCTion and GRAIL. Despite the prediction of 70 exons by DiCTion and the prediction of 118 exons by GRAIL, neither programs accurately predicted the complete exon structure of CD28, CTLA4 or ICOS. DiCTion did not predict any sequences encoding ICOS. Of the remaining predicted exons, two were localized to intron 1 of CD28, and one was predicted in intron 3 of both CTLA4 and ICOS receptor loci. Assuming that the predicted intronic exons are false positives, these results suggest that up to 56 potential DiCTion ORFs remain in this region of 381 kb. GRAIL analysis generated even more potential exons than DiCTion including some open reading frames containing CD28 (CDS-1, CDS-2, CDS-4), CTLA4 (CDS-2), and ICOS (CDS-1, CDS-2, CDS-4). In appearance, GRAIL was more successful in exon prediction, but closer analysis shows that GRAIL tended to overpredict exons more than DiCTion. For example, in the CD28 intron 1, GRAIL predicted 8 exons while DiCTion predicted 1 exon. Although it has been reported that CD28 may be expressed as alternatively spliced products (Lee et al., 1990), it has not been demonstrated that intronic sequences described here contribute to the final products of known isoform variants. When DiCTion and GRAIL outputs were compared, 13 exons were found in common to both. Of these, three correspond to the known sequences CD28 CDS-2, CTLA4 CDS-2 and EST M26697.

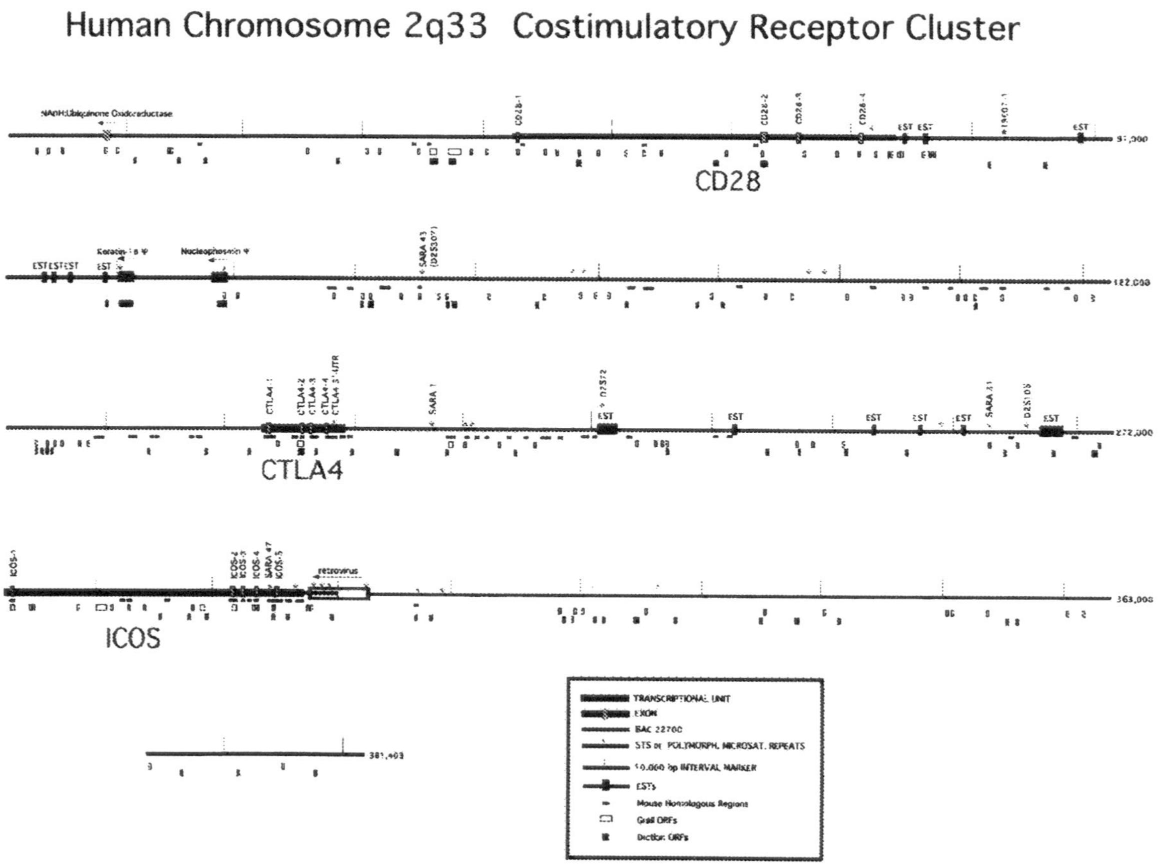

Human Chromosome 2q33 Costimulatory Receptor Cluster

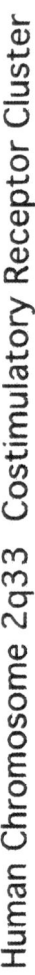

Figure 3. Annotated diagram of the the assembled 2q33 costimulatory receptor region.

90

Genomic Microarray Expression Analysis (GMEA):

The use of oligonucleotide and cDNA microarray technology has transformed the study of gene regulation from a focused examination of a few genes to a nearly comprehensive examination of the entire transcriptome. Both of these technologies, however, are limited by the need to correctly and comprehensively identify all transcribed genes. Genes that have not been identified by EST sequencing efforts or ab initio gene prediction programs cannot be monitored by these methods. We have developed the method of genomic microarray expression analysis (GMEA) to scan genomic DNA for differentially transcribed genes without the bias of gene predictions. Using this approach, genomic BAC clones used in this study, sheared to an average size of 2 kb, were subcloned to create libraries. Subclones from the BAC libraries were then PCR amplified and arrayed on glass slides to create genomic microarrays. Genomic regions from differentially transcribed genes were then identified after hybridization with total RNA from non-stimulated or PMA-ionomycin treated CD4+ T-cells.

In a pilot experiment we scanned 182 Kb of genomic sequence spanning the ICOS and CTLA4 loci for genes that are upregulated upon T-cell activation. Using the BAC 22700 subclone library, 620 sequence-characterized subclones were analyzed, resulting in 18 clones showing reproducible differential hybridization. Eight clones corresponded to sequences within the CTLA4 locus, 7 clones corresponded only to the ICOS 3' UTR and 3 clones corresponded to both ICOS 3' UTR and endogenous retroviral sequences immediately 3' of ICOS (Figure 4, Donor A+B). Differential hybridization detected to ICOS was to the region corresponding to the longest transcribed unit, the 2 kb 3' UTR. More importantly, it should be noted that the absence of other differentially hybridizing genomic fragments suggests that no other PMA-ionomycin activated T-cell genes are present within the 181,654 bp section between position 119,296 and 300,949 of the costimulatory receptor region.

To extend our search for nearby genes involved in T-cell activation, we scanned nearly all of the 381 Kb costimulatory receptor locus by including subclone libraries from BAC 22606 and BAC 22608. An additional 12 subclones mapping to ICOS were identified from BAC 22608, however, no other new clones showed differential expression. This was somewhat surprising since BAC 22606 spans CD28. Examination of subclone sequence and the DNA used for microarray fabrication revealed that two clones containing

CD28 sequence had been successfully arrayed. Both clones were detected above background in both untreated and PMA-ionomycin treated T-cells with no significant difference between the two samples. The lack of detected differential expression was most likely due to ALU sequences included in these two subclones masking any difference. Alternatively, the constitutively expressed CD28 gene was not sufficiently upregulated to be detected by the methods used here. The use of smaller subclones with more thorough coverage of the genomic region examined could help separate regions of repetitive sequence from simple coding sequence and allow genes with repetitive sequence to be detected by GMEA.

The use of differential expression as a means to identify gene of interest in genomic sequence has significant benefits as well as potential pitfalls. Repetitive sequence will be equally represented in most RNA samples, so clones containing repetitive sequence will generally fail to show differential expression. While this can mask real results, it has the significant benefit of limiting false positives.

Additional information about the location of genes within genomic sequence can possibly be derived from the absolute hybridization signal from both samples, even when no difference is detected. Of the 620 sequence derived from BAC 22700, hybridization significantly above background levels was detected from 287 clones. Many of these subclones map to regions with no predicted exon or repetitive sequence. Whether these clones actually contain novel genes that are present in both the experimental and reference samples or simply contain sequences showing cross hybridization remains to be determined.

With the recent release of the preliminary human genome sequence (Venter et al., 2001; McPherson et al., 2001), experimental approaches to identify and validate transcribed genes will be critical to our understanding of the transcriptome. One powerful approach of scanning the genome for exons couples ab initio gene prediction with experimental validation using microarrays. Using this approach, all 442,785 predicted exons from the available human genome sequence were placed onto a set of 50 arrays and used validate exons then join co-expressed exons into predicted genes (Shoemaker et al., 2001). These exon arrays will prove useful at validating exons predicted by ab initio programs, but do not provide any information about exons that were not predicted. The GMEA approach, with its independence from gene predictions, will be useful in identifying novel genes narrowly defined genomic regions, such as those generated in disease gene mapping studies or in regions containing gene clusters.

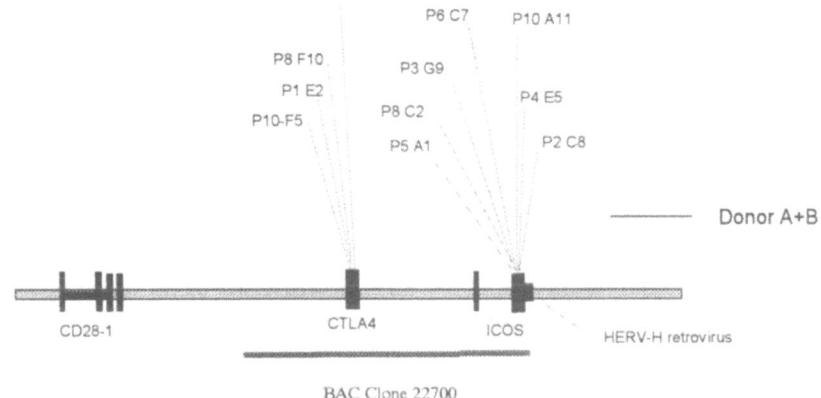

Figure 4. Genomic microarray expression analysis of the costimulatoryreceptor region. Location of of genomic sites corresponding to dfferentially hybridizing events are indicated.

2q33 HERV-H endogenous retrovirus: Natural occurrence of ICOS antisense transcripts

Analysis of the 2q33 HERV-H LTR in the region studied indicated that myb binding sites were present, suggesting these retroviral LTRs were poised for transcription initiation. From the data presented, it could not be determined whether hybridization to ICOS 3'-UTR and retroviral sequences detected by GMEA reflected transcription from the ICOS promoter or whether these differential hybridization signal reflected actual retroviral transcripts induced in PMA-ionomycin induced T-cells.

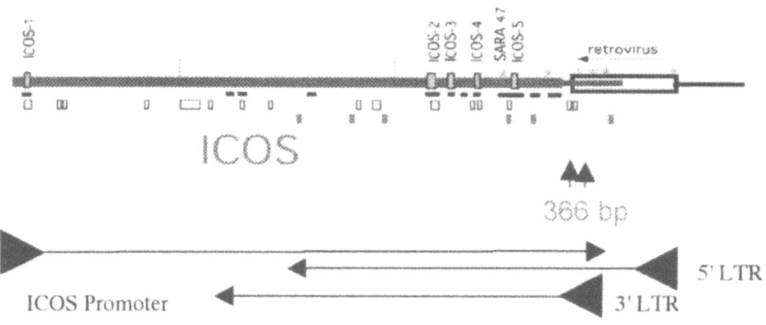

Figure 5. Potential transcription start sites flanking the ICOS gene.

Northern blots were performed to determine transcript orientation from this region (Figure 6). ICOS 3' UTR sequences were subcloned into T7-promoter bearing vectors in each orientation and used to generate strand-specific radiolabeled probes. RNA from two donor CD4+ T-cells and Jurkat T-cell line preparations, cultured either in the presence or the absence of PMA-ionomycin activation, were fractionated, blotted and hybridized to either the ICOS sense or antisense probe. With the ICOS antisense probe, a discrete hybridization signal was observed for activated samples but not for non-activated samples, corroborating previous reports of ICOS being an inducible costimulatory molecule. Hybridization with ICOS sense probe also signal, indicating the presence of antisense ICOS transcripts. Two regions of clear hybridization signals were detected in all samples examined; one discrete band at approximately 6.5 kb and one non-discrete band at ~3-4 kb. These results strongly suggest that the retroviral LTR promoters 3' of ICOS are transcriptionally active and at least one set are responsive to cell activation. The 6 kb band appeared to be preferentially induced on activated CD4+ T-cells while being constitutively expressed in both Jurkat cells samples. The 3-4 kb band appeared to be expressed in all samples examined regardless of activation state. Because these retroviral transcripts may be derived from either the 5' LTR or the 3' LTR viral promoter, two potential sets of transcripts may be detected, which is reflected in the data presented. Examination of sequences within 7.5

kb upstream from the ICOS 3' UTR revealed the presence of 8 cannonical polyadenylation signals (AATAAA), suggesting that LTR driven transcription may result in multiple transcript sizes as reflected in the non-discrete 3-4 kb hybridization bands.

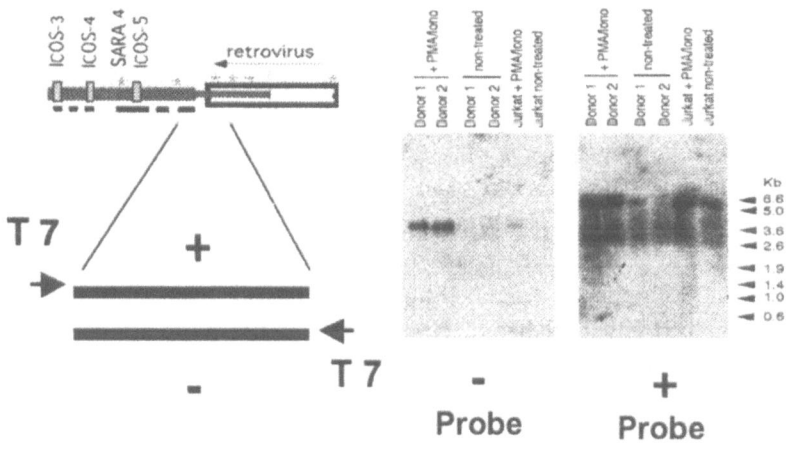

Figure 6. Strand specific hybridization of ICOS 3'-UTR to activated versus non-activated T-cell RNA.

The retroviral 3'-LTR to ICOS 3' UTR amplification product is obtained from a diverse panel of human genomic DNA suggesting the presence of this HERV-H is widely distributed. The retroviral transcription found here is consistent with reports by reporter gene assays demonstrating certain HERV-H LTRs function as transcriptionally active promoters with dependency on myb (de Parseval et al., 1999) and sp1 (Sjottem et al., 1996) transcription factors. Thus, it is possible that biological events such as mutations or gene rearrangements, may lead to the alteration of HERV-H LTR promoter activity and produce antisense ICOS transcripts and formation of RNAi (Zamore et al., 2000) that could destabilize normal ICOS transcription. Of the cytokine panel that is elicited by ICOS receptor signaling in T-cell activation assays, superinduction of the Th-2 cytokine IL-10 appears to the most prominent (Hutloff et al., 1999) although IL-4, IL-5, gamma-IFN, TNF alpha and GM-CSF were also produced. Given the complex nature of this cytokine panel, alteration of

ICOS signaling could potentiate cytokine skewing and deviate T-cell function. Indeed, indirect evidence suggest that endogenous retroviral genes are linked with numerous autoimmune diseases such as systemic lupus erythematosus, multiple sclerosis, type I diabetes, and Sjogren's syndrome (Mason et al., 1999; Nakagawa and Harrison, 1996). Mechanisms have been proposed by which endogenous retroviruses lead to immune dysregulation. Retroviral cis-regulatory elements may influence transcription of cellular genes involved in immune function, whereas retroviral transactivating elements, like tax in human T-lymphotrophic virus type I or tat in human immunodeficiency virus-I, may induce cellular genes not necessarily proximal to the retroviral element. Indeed, transient upregulation of ICOS receptor [H4] surface display has been reported to be associated with the early phase of HIV infection and with gradual increase during disease progression (Lucia et al., 2000). Whether ICOS gene transcription is regulated by HIV or any other retrovirus remains to be determined. Further studies of the biological activity of HERV-H endogenous retrovirus in relation to ICOS transcriptional stability may allow greater insight on whether cytokine balance in immunological disease is linked to this specific region of DNA.

Additional polymorphic microsatellite markers permits reassessment of CTLA4 linkage to genetic diseases

To identify additional markers in this region that may also serve to refine the associations between genetic diseases and the costimulatory receptor region of 2q33, 25 microsatellite repeat sequences in the BAC 22700 clone were analyzed for the presence of repeat unit polymorphisms. Among the 25 repeats examined, genomic DNA PCR amplification of a panel of 13 individuals revealed 4 polymorphic microsatellites, corresponding to di-, tri- and hexanucleotide repeats. Of the 4 polymorphic microsatellite repeats examined (Figure 2), repeat SARA 31(nt. 263,177-263,211; [ATTTTTT]n6) was represented by 2 alleles, repeat SARA 1(nt. 217,444-217,492; [TATC]n12) was represented by 4 alleles, while SARA 43 (nt. 125,845-125,892 [GT]n24, later found to be homologous to sequences within D2S307) and SARA 47 (nt. 295,275-295,326; [GT]n15) appeared to be highly polymorphic with greater than 6 different alleles within 13 individuals examined. Analysis of the 13 individuals for the polymorphisms associated with the known CTLA4 3' UTR (nt. 209,177-209,216; [AT]n40) microsatellite repeat demonstrated 2 alleles. Compilation and comparison of the 4 polymorphic microsatellite alleles found in these individuals revealed no shared allelic combination, suggesting that this set of 4 polymorphic markers in combination with existing markers, may be effectively applied to haplotype determination and the high resolution discrimination of genetic associations of disease states linked to the costimulatory receptor region.

The close proximity of the ICOS locus to CTLA4 raises the possibility that genetic linkage of human autoimmune diseases to 2q33 could be due to variants in the ICOS locus, rather than the CD28 or CTLA4 loci. Chronic stimulation of ICOS receptor in ICOS-ligand transgenic mice revealed a phenotype consistent with B-cell hyperstimulation (Yoshinaga et al., 1999). Grave's disease and type 1 diabetes share etiology in which autoimmune antibodies are generated, suggesting a dysregulation of B cell differentiation and antibody production. A recent genetic study using STS located within 200 Kb of CTLA4 revealed a high level of linkage disequilibrium with the onset of type 1 diabetes as reflected by the genetic locus IDDM12 (Marron et al., 2000). Because of the limited coverage obtained from the number of markers used, the authors concluded that IDDM12 exists within roughly 100 kb of CTLA4 locus but is not CD28. However, the IDDM12 physical map used in that study is not in agreement with the sequence presented here; the IDDM12 physical map suggests the markers occur in the order 19E07, D2S307, D2S72, CTLA4, D2S105 whereas the sequence presented here indicates the order 19E07, D2S307, CTLA4, D2S72, D2S105, ICOS (Figure 7). The region of linkage disequilibrium may thus be shifted downstream from CTLA4 towards ICOS, leaving open the possibility that the regions near ICOS are linked to the IDDM12 locus, especially when the distance between the ICOS and CTLA4 loci is less than 100 kb.

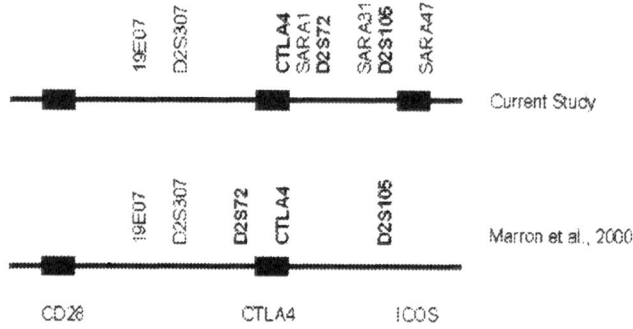

Figure 7. Comparison of polymorphic microsatellite sites determined in current sequence assembly and those from prior 2q33 mapping study.

To generate a higher resolution map diagnostic for genetic diseases, we examined 5 microsatellite repeats SARA 31, CTLA4 3' UTR, SARA 1, SARA 43 (D2S307), and SARA 47 periodically located at approximately 50 kb intervals between CD28 and ICOS (Figure 2). These markers revealed polymorphisms that are not linked in terms of allelic variation patterning. Most notably, the ICOS intron 4 SARA 47 microsatellite repeat may prove useful as a polymorphic marker in genetic studies. SARA 47 showed extreme variation with at least 6 different alleles with no two identical allelic patterning within the random group of 13 individuals. Beyond the microsatellites ana-lyzed, we identified an additional 348 simple repetitive elements comprising 2.5% of the total region, but have not yet determined the polymorphic state of these sites.

The complete assembly of the costimulatory receptor region sets the foundation for the high resolution discrimination of genetic disease association to numerous elements within this region by the use of the representative panel of microsatellite repeats described here or by the future elucidation of SNPs at desired locations. The future genetic analysis of these polymorphisms within patient populations in combination with GMEA of 2q33 and other regions, flow cytometric analysis of each receptor to determine the regulation surface protein display, and RNA analysis of potential anti-sense transcripts, will point to the identification of the true genomic element(s) contributing to autoimmune disease.

References

1. Abbas, A. K., and Sharpe, A. H (1999) T-cell stimulation: an abundance of B7s [news; comment]. Nat Med 5: 1345-6.
2. Aicher, A., Hayden-Ledbetter, M., Brady, W. A., Pezzutto, A., Richter, G., Magaletti, D., Buckwalter, S., Ledbetter, J. A. and Clark, E. A. (2000) Characterization of human inducible costimulator ligand expression and function. J Immunol 164: 4689-96.
3. Balzano, C., Buonavista, N., Rouvier, E. and Golstein, P (1992) CTLA-4 and CD28: similar proteins, neighbouring genes. Int J Cancer Suppl 7: 28-32.
4. de Parseval, N., Alkabbani, H. and Heidmann, T (1999) The long terminal repeats of the HERV-H human endogenous retrovirus contain binding sites for transcriptional regulation by the Myb protein. J Gen Virol 80: 841-5.
5. Deng, Z., Haghighi, F., Helleby, L., Vanterpool, K., Horn, E. M., Barst, R. J., Hodge, S. E., Morse, J. H. and Knowles, J. A (2000a) Fine mapping of PPH1, a gene for familial primary pulmonary hypertension, to a 3-cM region on chromosome 2q33. Am J Respir Crit Care Med 161: 1055-9.
6. Deng, Z., Morse, J. H., Slager, S. L., Cuervo, N., Moore, K. J., Venetos, G., Kalachikov, S., Cayanis, E., Fischer, S. G., Barst, R. J., Hodge, S. E. and Knowles, J. A (2000b) Familial Primary Pulmonary Hypertension (Gene PPH1) Is Caused by Mutations in the Bone Morphogenetic Protein Receptor-II Gene. Am J Hum Genet 67.
7. Dong H., Zhu G., Tamada K., and Chen L (1999) B7-H1, a third member of the B7 family, co-stimulates T-cell proliferation and interleukin-10 secretion. Nat Med 1999 Dec;5(12):1365-9
8. Finger, L. R., Pu, J., Wasserman, R., Vibhakar, R., Louie, E., Hardy, R. R., Burrows, P. D., and Billips, L. G (1997) The human PD-1 gene: complete cDNA, genomic organization, and developmentally regulated expression in B cell progenitors. Gene 197:177-187.

9. Freeman, G. J., Long, A. J., Iwai, Y., Latchman, Y., Bourque, K., Chernova, T., Nishimura, H., Fitz, L. J., Malenkovich, N., Okazaki, T., Byrne, M. C., Horton, H. F., Fouser, L., Carter, L., Ling, V., Bowman, M. R., Sharpe, A. H., Carreno, B. M., Collins, M., Wood, C. R., and Honjo, T (2000) Engagement of the PD-1 immunoinhibitory receptor by a novel B7-family member leads to negative regulation of lymphocyte activation. Journal of Experimental Medicine 192:1024-1034.

10. Frazer, K. A., Ueda, Y., Zhu, Y., Gifford, V. R., Garofalo, M. R., Mohandas, N., Martin, C. H., Palazzolo, M. J., Cheng, J. F. and Rubin, E. M (1997) Computational and biological analysis of 680 kb of DNA sequence from the human 5q31 cytokine gene cluster region. Genome Res 7: 495-512.

11. Hattori, M., Fujiyama, A., Taylor, T. D., Watanabe, H., Yada, T., Park, H. S., Toyoda, A., Ishii, K., Totoki, Y., Choi, D. K., Soeda, E., Ohki, M., Takagi, T., Sakaki, Y., Taudien, S., Blechschmidt, K., Polley, A., Menzel, U., Delabar, J., Kumpf, K., Lehmann, R., Patterson, D., Reichwald, K., Rump, A., Schillhabel, M. and Schudy, A. (2000) The DNA sequence of human chromosome 21. The chromosome 21 mapping and sequencing consortium [see comments]. Nature 405: 311-9.

12. Hutloff, A., Dittrich, A. M., Beier, K. C., Eljaschewitsch, B., Kraft, R., Anagnostopoulos, I. and Kroczek, R. A (1999) ICOS is an inducible T-cell co-stimulator structurally and functionally related to CD28. Nature 397: 263-6.

13. Kristiansen, O.P., Larsen Z.M., and Pociot, F (2000) CTLA-4 in autoimmune diseases - a general susceptibility gene to autoimmunity? Genes and Immunity 1:170-184.

14. Kim, J. W., Lee, Y., Kang, H. B., Chose, Y. K., Chung, T. W., Chang, S. Y., Lee, K. S. and Choe, I. S (1997) Cloning of the human cDNA sequence encoding the NADH:ubiquinone oxidoreductase MLRQ subunit. Biochem Mol Biol Int 43: 669-75.

15. Lee, K. P., Taylor, C., Petryniak, B., Turka, L. A., June, C. H. and Thompson, C. B (1990) The genomic organization of the CD28 gene. Implications for the regulation of CD28 mRNA expression and heterogeneity. J Immunol 145: 344-52.

16. Ling, V., Wu, P. W., Finnerty, H. F., Bean, K. M., Spaulding, V., Fouser, L. A., Leonard, J. P., Hunter, S. E., Zollner, R., Thomas, J.

L., Miyashiro, J. S., Jacobs, K. A. and Collins, M (2000) Cutting edge: identification of GL50, a novel B7-like protein that functionally binds to ICOS receptor. J Immunol 164: 1653-7.

17. Ling, V., Wu, P. W., Finnerty, H. F., Sharpe, A. H., Gray, G. S. and Collins, M (1999) Complete Sequence Determination of the Mouse and Human CTLA4 Gene Loci: Cross-Species DNA Sequence Similarity beyond Exon Borders. Genomics 60: 341-355.

18. Ling, V., Wu, P. W., Finnerty, H. F., Agostino, M. J., Graham, J. R, Chen, S., Jussiff J. M., Fisk G. J., Miller, C. P., and Collins, M.. Assembly and annotation of human chromosome 2q33 sequence containing the CD28, CTLA4 and ICOS gene cluster: Analysis by computational, comparative and microarray approaches. Genomics (in press).

19. Lucia M. B., Buonfiglio D., Bottarel F., Bensi T., Rutella S., Rumi C., Ortona L., Janeway C. A. Jr, Cauda R., and Dianzani U (2000) Expression of the novel T cell activation molecule hpH4 in HIV-infected patients: correlation with disease status. AIDS Res. Hum. Retroviruses 16:549-57

20. M Pherson, J. D., et al., The International Human Mapping Consortium. A physical map of the human genome. Nature 409:816-8.

21. Marron, M. P., Zeidler, A., Raffel, L. J., Eckenrode, S. E., Yang, J. J., Hopkins, D. I., Garchon, H. J., Jacob, C. O., Serrano-Rios, M., Martinez Larrad, M. T., Park, Y., Bach, J. F., Rotter, J. I., Yang, M. C. and She, J. X (2000) Genetic and physical mapping of a type 1 diabetes susceptibility gene (IDDM12) to a 100-kb phagemid artificial chromosome clone containing D2S72-CTLA4-D2S105 on chromosome 2q33. Diabetes 49: 492-9.

22. Mason, A. L., Xu, L., Guo, L. and Garry, R. F (1999) Retroviruses in autoimmune liver disease: genetic or environmental agents? Arch Immunol Ther Exp (Warsz) 47: 289-97.

23. Nakagawa, K., and Harrison, L. C (1996) The potential roles of endogenous retroviruses in autoimmunity. Immunol Rev 152: 193-236.

24. Oshima, R. G., Baribault, H. and Caulin, C (1996) Oncogenic regulation and function of keratins 8 and 18. Cancer Metastasis Rev 15: 445-71.

25. Philpott, A., Krude, T. and Laskey, R. A (2000) Nuclear chaperones. Semin Cell Dev Biol 11: 7-14.

26. Sansom, D. M (2000) CD28, CTLA-4 and their ligands: who does what and to whom? Immunology 101:169-177.

27. Sjottem, E., Anderssen, S. and Johansen, T (1996) The promoter activity of long terminal repeats of the HERV-H family of human retrovirus-like elements is critically dependent on Sp1 family proteins interacting with a GC/GT box located immediately 3' to the TATA box. J Virol 70: 188-98.

28. Yoshinaga, S. K., Whoriskey, J. S., Khare, S. D., Sarmiento, U., Guo, J., Horan, T., Shih, G., Zhang, M., Coccia, M. A., Kohno, T., Tafuri-Bladt, A., Brankow, D., Campbell, P., Chang, D., Chiu, L., Dai, T., Duncan, G., Elliott, G. S., Hui, A., McCabe, S. M., Scully, S., Shahinian, A., Shaklee, C. L., Van, G., Mak, T. W. and et al (1999) T-cell co-stimulation through B7RP-1 and ICOS. Nature 402: 827-32.

29. Venter JC, et al. Celera Genomics (2001) The sequence of the human genome. Science 16:1304-1351.

30. Ward, S. G. (1996) CD28: a signalling perspective. Biochem J 318:361-77.

31. Zamore, P. D., Tuschl, T., Sharp, P. A. and Bartel, D. P (2000) RNAi: double-stranded RNA directs the ATP-dependent cleavage of mRNA at 21 to 23 nucleotide intervals. Cell 101: 25-33.

CTLA-4 gene in the pathogenesis of Graves' disease

Tatsuo Yanagawa, Tsuyoshi Kouki* and Leslie J DeGroot*

Department of Medicine, Nerima General Hospital, Tokyo, Japan; and *Thyroid Study Unit, Department of Medicine, University of Chicago, Chicago, IL 60637, USA

Address all correspondence and requests for reprints to:

Tatsuo Yanagawa, M.D., PhD.: Department of Medicine, Nerima General Hospital 2-41-1 Asahigaoka, Nerima-ku, Tokyo 176-8530, Japan

TEL: 81-3-3972-1001, Fax: 81-3-3972-1031

E-mail : VZA07472@nifty.ne.jp

Introduction

There is growing evidence that CTLA-4 is an important susceptibility gene in Graves' disease (GD), as well as in many other autoimmne diseases. We have the honor of being pioneers in this field, and our data and others are presented in this paper.

Key words

CTLA-4, Graves' disease, autoimmune thyroid disease, HLA, DQA1*0501, CD28, diabetes

HLA and GD

GD is an autoimmune thyroid disease, characterized by the production of TSH receptor autoantibodies that cause hyperthyroidism. Like many other autoimmune diseases, GD is associated with specific HLA genes.

Ealier studies in 1970's, revealed that HLA-B8 is associated with GD in caucasians. In 1980's, the association of GD was found to be stronger with HLA-DR3 than with HLA-B8. The relative risk, however, remained weak, and led us to a search for association with other HLA alleles, using the PCR-SSO method (1).

HLA-DQA1*0501 was found to be positively associated with GD. The frequency of HLA-DR3 is higher and HLA-DQA1*0201 lower in GD patients, but the differences did not reach statistical significance. Most subsequent studies revealed similar results. We also proposed that the association of GD with DQA1*0501 is independent of DR3 (1), and that it may be stronger in males (2). However there is no consensus on this point.

Time to focus on chromosomal loci other than HLA

Potential associations have been sought between GD and non-HLA markers. Unfortunately, studies of other genes for association with GD have not been informative and have often produced conflicting results. In 1994, it was time to focus on chromosomal loci other than HLA (3). We therefore examined several candidate genes that are directly related to autoimmunity or encode thyroid antigens, including the cytotoxic T lymphocyte antigen-4 (CTLA-4) gene (4).

Why CTLA-4 gene?

Antigen specific T cell activation involves at least two signals: one mediated by interaction of the T cell receptor with a specific antigen in association with HLA molecules, and the second, an antigen-independent, costimulatory signal, provided by the interaction of CD28 on T cells and the B7 family (CD80, CD86) on antigen-presenting cells. CTLA-4 is another ligand for B7. CTLA-4 is expressed on activated T cells, and terminates T-cell activation by binding to B7 family. It plays an essential role in the establishment of peripheral self-tolerance as well as the regulation of normal T-cell immunity (5). In 1994, it was not known whether the CTLA-4 molecule deliver either positive or negative signals to T cells. In either way, we believed that CTLA-4 should be a key molecule in controlling the immune response because it is expressed only when T cells are activated. We therefore examined the association between CTLA-4 gene and GD, and were excited by the results (4).

Genotype frequencies of CTLA-4 alleles in patients with GD and controls

The polymorphic AT repeats are in the 3' untranslated region of exon 4 of the human CTLA-4 gene on chromosome 2.   Twenty-one alleles were observed with sizes ranging from 88-134 base pairs.   In the association analysis, the genotype frequencies between GD patients and controls differed significantly ($P = 0.012$), and the difference was attributable to a higher frequency of the 106-basepair allele among patients (relative risk, 2.82).   When the patients were subdivided with respect to sex and HLA, the phenotype frequencies of allele 106 was higher in the female patients with protective HLA specificities (DQA1*0201 positive/DQA1*0501 negative) than in those with susceptible HLA specificities (DQA1*0201 negative/DQA1*0501 positive; 81.8% vs. 45.5%; $P = 0.026$). The CTLA-4 gene or a closely associated gene (including CD28) confers susceptibility to GD.   This association may be more important in female patients with protective HLA specificities, who otherwise would be at low risk of developing the disease.

CTLA-4 gene, as a major GD locus

Many studies supported the association of CTLA-4 gene with GD, by studying the three polymorphisms in the CTLA-4 locus: the microsatellite (AT)n repeat in the 3' untranslated region, an A/G transition in position 49 of exon 1, and a C to T transition at position -318 of the promoter sequence.   The G allele in exon 1 and 106bp AT repeat allele in exon 4 are in tight linkage disequilibrium with each other.   A recent genetic linkage study has demonstrated CTLA-4 as a major GD susceptibility locus.   The CTLA-4 locus confers 29-34% of the total genetic susceptibility to GD and HLA region confers 17-20% in an UK Caucasian population (6).

CTLA-4 and various autoimmune diseases

Subsequent studies revealed the association with various autoimmune diseases (7), such as Hashimoto's thyroiditis, type 1 diabetes, Addison's disease, multiple sclerosis, myasthenia gravis, and Celiac disease.   It is unclear whether CTLA-4 gene itself confers susceptibility, or these alleles serve as markers for variation in the coding or regulatory regions of the CTLA-4 gene, CD28 gene, or unknown gene in linkage disequilibrium with CTLA-4 gene. Recent studies narrowed the type 1 diabetes susceptibility interval to a 100 Kb genomic region (8).   It is likely that CTLA-4 gene itself confers susceptibility to type 1 diabetes and possibly to other autoimmune diseases.

CTLA-4 gene polymorphisms and T cell function

It is not clear how CTLA-4 gene polymorphism contributes to the pathogenesis of autoimmune diseases. The associations between CTLA-4 gene polymorophisms and T cell function have been investigated by us and others. Length of the AT repeat in exon 4 is potentially important because it may be involved in mRNA stability (4). A study by Huang et al. showed that alleles with longer PCR products in an (AT)n polymorphism in CTLA-4 lead to T cell hyper-reactivity (9).

We found that the position 49A/G alleleism in exon 1 of the leader sequence affects the function of the CTLA-4 gene products. The G allele is associated with less inhibition of T cell proliferation, which is uncovered when the CTLA-4 signal is blocked (10). This difference in function is not specific for GD but exists in all subjects with the G allele. Thus the HLA association provides a disease-specific hightened risk for GD, and the CTLA-4 allelism provide a modest non-specific augmentation of immune reactivity which can increase risk for many autoimmune diseases. It is conceivable that differences in the leader sequence of the gene may result in altered rates of endocytosis or surface trafficking, or that the effect is actually through the 3' AT repeat allelism, which is tightly linked. Further studies are necessary to understand the regulation of T-cell mediated immune responses, which may influence the pathogenesis of autoimmune diseases.

Concluding remarks

CTLA-4 gene region has been established as a susceptibility loci for GD, and the functional significance of CTLA-4 gene polymorphism has been elucidated. Several loci other than HLA and CTLA-4 have been suggested as GD susceptibility genes, but confirmation of the importance of these loci is lacking. Additional loci are likely to be identified via a combination of genome-wide linkage analysis and allelic association analysis of candidate genes. Now it is time to identify the full genetic susceptibility to GD.

References

1. Yanagawa T, Mangklabruks A, Chang YB, Okamoto Y, Fisfalen ME, Curran PG, DeGroot LJ (1993) Human histocompatibility leukocyte antigen-DQA1*0501 allele associated with genetic susceptibility to Graves'

disease in a caucasian population.   J Clin Endocrinol Metab 76:1569-1574.

2.   Yanagawa T, Mangklabruks A, DeGroot LJ (1994) Strong association between HLA-DQA1*0501 and Graves' disease in a male caucasian population.   J Clin Endocrinol Metab 79:227-229.

3.   McLachlan SM (1993) Editorial: the genetic basis of autoimmune thyroid disease: time to focus on chromosomal loci other than the major histocompatibility complex (HLA in men). J Clin Endocrinol Metab 77:605A-605C.

4.   Yanagawa T, Hidaka Y, Guimaraes V, Soliman M, DeGroot LJ (1995) CTLA-4 gene polymorphism associated with Graves' disease in a caucasian population.   J Clin Endocrinol Metab 80:41-45.

5.   Thompson CB, Allison JP (1997) The emerging role of CTLA-4 as immune attenuator.   Immunity 7:445-450.

6.   Vaidya B, Imrie H, Perros P, Young ET, Kelly WF, Carr D, Large DM, Toft AD, McCarthy MI, Kendall-Taylor P, Pearce SH (1999) The cytotoxic T lymphocyte antigen-4 is a major Graves' disease locus. Hum Mol Genet 8:1195-1199.

7.   Kristiansen OP, Larsen ZM, Pociot F (2000) CTLA-4 in autoimmune diseases--a general susceptibility gene to autoimmunity? Genes Immun 1:170-184.

8.   Marron MP, Zeidler A, Raffel LJ, Eckenrode SE, Yang JJ, Hopkins DI, Garchon HJ, Jacob CO, Serrano-Rios M, Larrad MTM, Park Y, Bach JF, Rotter JI, Yang MCK, She JX (2000) Genetic and physical mapping of a type 1 diabetes susceptibility gene (IDDM12) to a 100-Kb phagimid artificial chromosome clone containing D2S72-CTLA4-D2S105 on chromosome 2q33. Diabetes 49:492-499.

9.   Huang D, Giscombe R, Zhou Y, Pirskanen R, Lefvert AK (2000) Dinucleotide repeat expansion in the CTLA-4 gene leads to T cell hyperreactivity via the CD28 pathway in myasthenia gravis. J Neuroimmunology 105:69-77.

10.   Kouki T, Sawai Y, Gardine CA, Fisfalen ME, Alegre ML, DeGroot LJ (2000)   CTLA-4 gene polymorphism at position 49 in exon 1 reduces the inhibitory function of CTLA-4 and contributes to the pathogenesis of Graves' disease. J Immunol 165:6606-6611.

The evolving role of CTLA-4 in the genetic predisposition to AITD

Giuseppe Barbesino, MD
Department of Endocrinology University of Pisa, Pisa, Italy
Via Paradisa 2 56124 PISA-ITALY E-mail: gbarbe@tiscalinet.it

Introduction

The autoimmune thyroid diseases (AITD), Graves' diseases (GD) and Hashimoto's thyroiditis (HT) show a clear genetic component in epidemiological studies. The search for the genes responsible for the inheritance of the AITD has since many years provided evidence that some HLA haplotypes give a small, although significant contribution to the genetic susceptibility to the disease. Recently, the developments of the human genome-mapping project have provided the tools for whole genome scans. While this approach has yielded a number of loci of interest, precise definition of the genes at these loci is till under way. But the genome mapping efforts has also provided information on a number of new candidate genes, mainly immune response genes and thyroid autoantigens, that have been studied in both association and linkage studies for a possible involvement in AITD. To date only the cytotoxic T-lymphocyte antigen-4 (CTLA-4) gene has emerged consistently as a second contributor to the genetic susceptibility to the AITD. CTLA-4 is an important down-regulator of the immune response and represents therefore an excellent candidate for autoimmunity. In this paper the current evidence for an involvement of the CTLA-4 gene in the genetic predisposition to AITD will be reviewed.

Key Words

autoimmune thyroid diseases, Graves' diseases, Hashimoto's thyroiditis, HLA, CTLA-4, CD28, ICOS, B7

The role of CTLA-4 and related genes in the regulation of the immune response

The human CTLA-4 gene product is a protein of the immunoglobulin gene superfamily. The CTLA-4 molecule is a transmembrane receptor of approximately 40 Kda (1). CTLA-4 shares considerable homology with CD28 (2) and the recently described inducible co-stimulator (ICOS) genes (3). CTLA-4 is also similar to synthenic proteins of other mammalians (1), indicating preservation along the evolutionary line. The CTLA-4 gene has been mapped to chromosome 2q33 (4), only 25 to 150 kb apart from the CD28 gene (2) and also close to the Inducible Co-stimulator (ICOS) gene (5). The chromosomal proximity of CTLA4, CD28 and ICOS and their close homology suggest that these genes evolved, possibly by duplication, from a common ancestor gene. While CD28 is constitutively expressed on T-cells, the CTLA-4 and ICOS gene are expressed on T-cells only after antigen or mythogen stimulation (6). Both CTLA-4 and CD28 interact with B7 molecules expressed on antigen-presenting cells (APC). However, while the CD28-B7 interaction leads to T-cell activation and proliferation, the subsequent expression of CTLA-4 leads to a higher affinity CTLA-4-B7 interaction, which eventually silences or kills activated T-cells (7). Therefore, CTLA-4 acts as key down-regulator of the immune response and represents an excellent candidate as an autoimmunity gene. Animal models underscore the importance of these mechanisms in the physiologic control of the immune response. Mice defective in CTLA-4 function (CTLA-4 -/-) develop a rapidly fatal disease, with multiorgan lymphocytic infiltrates, which is a striking counterpart of human autoimmune diseases (8). Similarly to CTLA-4, ICOS is only expressed on activated T-cells, after co-stimulation via the CD28-B7 pathway (5). The ligand of ICOS on presenting cells has been named ICOS-L or B7-H2 and is homologous but different from B7 (5). The interaction of ICOS with its ligand induces T-cell proliferation and secretion of a number of cytokines, such as IL-4, IL-5, IL-6, IFN-γ, TNF-α (3). ICOS is therefore probably involved in the amplification of the secondary immune response. In summary, the chromosomal region 2q33-34 contains at least three (and possibly more) important immune regulatory genes, which represent important candidates for the genetic predisposition to autoimmunity. With this respect, the CTLA-4 gene has been studied in greater detail, but the close genetic proximity of these three genes must be taken into account when interpreting genetic data obtained with classical methods (linkage and association). Indeed, positive linkage or association data obtained with markers in this region may well indicate that any of these three genes are involved in the genetic predisposition to AITD, unless very powerful datasets are studied or functional studies of variations in the three genes are performed.

Association studies of CTLA-4 in AITD

There are at least three well characterized polymorphic markers within or close to the CTLA-4 gene and these have been used in association studies to test the CTLA-4 gene as a candidate predisposing gene in AITD. The first described allelic system is a typical microsatellite marker, located in the 3' untranslated region of exon 3 of the gene. Amplification of this region by PCR with specific primers yields fragments of variable length, depending on the number of AT repeats contained in each allele (9). Using this marker, association of Graves' disease with CTLA-4 was first described by Yanagawa and colleagues. The 106 bp allele was found in about 27% of Graves' disease chromosomes from Caucasian patients, as compared with 14% of controls, yielding a relative risk of 2.82 (10). The 88 bp allele was the most represented allele (about 50% of control chromosomes) but there were at least twenty more alleles with very low prevalence in both controls and patients, preventing any further analysis. Other studies using this marker have confirmed an association of GD with the CTLA-4 106 bp in HT, but not with GD in a Japanese population (11). Because of the limitation of using very polymorphic markers in association studies, subsequent studies have employed single nucleotide polymorphisms (SNP), which are less polymorphic and therefore more useful in association studies. Two SNPs are known within the CTLA-4 gene. The first polymorphism is a A to G transition at position 49 of the coding sequence, causing a Threonine/Alanine substitution at codon 17 of the protein. Interestingly, the G allele shows strong (albeit incomplete) linkage disequilibrium with the 106 bp allele of the CTLA-4 microsatellite marker (12). It therefore represents an excellent substitute to the latter marker for association studies. Indeed the G allele has been shown to be associated with GD (12-17), HT (11, 16, 18) and even post-partum thyroiditis (19) in a number of studies, mostly in Caucasian and Asian populations (Figure 1). Only two negative studies are available in the literature in GD, in African Americans (20) and in HT in an Italian population (21). These differences may be attributed to different inclusion criteria, but it is possible that other loci or other alleles at the CTLA-4 locus have a role in different ethnic groups. Similarly to the microsatellite marker, this SNP yields small relative risks in AITD (Figure 1), indicating a small, albeit significant role of CTLA-4 in the genetic predisposition to AITD.

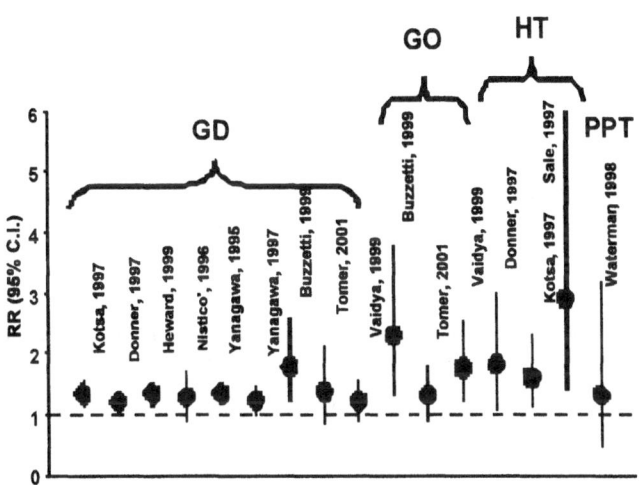

Figure 1. Association studies of CTLA-4 and AITD. Relative risks and 95% C.I. for the presence of the G allele of the 49 A/G CTLA-4 SNP are shown. GD= Graves' disease; GO=Graves' ophthalmopathy, HT, Hashimoto's thyroiditis, PPT, post-partum thyroiditis.

In spite of the high prevalence of the G allele in the general populations (therefore with a high prevalence of homozygosity), it is difficult to derive from available studies whether the homozygous state confers an additional risk as compared with heterozygosity. However, examining the available data, this doesn't seem to be the case and the effect of the G allele appears to be dominant. It must be remarked that the prevalence of the G allele varies significantly in different ethnic groups. The G allele is present in about 85% of Japanese controls and in 60% of Caucasian controls (Figure 2). These data underscore the need for careful selection of controls, since admixture of populations with different prevalence of the polymorphism and of the disease could cause falsely positive weak associations, through population stratification. It is also interesting to note that, because of the higher prevalence of the G allele in the Japanese population, one would expect a higher prevalence of AITD in this ethnic group. However, reliable comparative studies with this respect are very difficult to perform because of the confounding influence of environmental factors such as iodine intake and others and are not available to date.

In a few studies, the 49 A/G polymorphism has been studied in relation Graves' ophthalmopathy. Two studies reported a significant increase in the prevalence of the G allele in GD patients with ophthalmopathy as compared to GD patients without clinically relevant eye disease, in a British and an Italian population. In the first study the association was independent of the sex and of known environmental factors such as smoking or radioiodine treatment (22, 23). The second study confirmed the association of the G allele (in both the heterozygous and homozygous state) with Graves' ophthalmopathy, although, possibly because of the small size of the study, these authors were not able to confirm an association of the A/G polymorphism in GD patients without ophthalmopathy. We have recently addressed the problem of the genetic basis of Graves' ophthalmopathy from two different angles. In a segregation analysis of families of patients with Graves' ophthalmopathy we have sought evidence for a heritable factor responsible for Graves' ophthalmopathy per se and independent of the genetic predisposition to GD or AITD. Our analysis failed to show any influence of a genetic predisposition to Graves' ophthalmopathy per se (segregation ratio for Graves' ophthalmopathy: 0), while confirmed an increased risk for GD in first degree relatives of GD patients. Indeed, in keeping with these findings, the A/G polymorphism was associated with GD in our cohort, independently of the presence or absence of severe ophthalmopathy (24). We conclude therefore that it is likely that environmental factors play a major role in the pathogenesis of Graves' ophthalmopathy, in agreement with previous studies indicating at least two such factors: cigarette smoking and radioiodine (25).

Interestingly, the G allele has been associated to a variety of other autoimmune disorder, raising some questions on the specificity of these findings (26-32), Table 1.

112

Table 1. Selected association studies of CTLA-4 with various autoimmune disease.

Disease	RR	Marker	Reference
Primary biliary cirrhosis	2.45	49G	Agarwal, 2000
Autoimmune hepatitis	1.35	49G	Agarwal, 2000
IDDM	>4.7	49G	Awata, 1998
Coeliac disease	2.36	49A	Dijali-Saiah, 1999
Addison	1.7	49G	Donner, 1997
IDDM	1.4	49G	Donner, 1997
Vitiligo+AITD	3.2	106bp	Kemp, 1999
IDDM	2.13	49G	Lee, 2000
Rheumatoid arthritis	2.77	49G+HLA	Matsushita, 1999
IDDM	1.5	49G	Van Auwera,1999

The third known polymorphism of the CTLA-4 gene is a C to T (C/T) (SNP) transition at position –318 with respect to the start codon of the gene, which can be easily detected by RFLP analysis (33). This polymorphism has been studied in GD and HT Caucasian and Chinese populations. One study reported a significant association of the C allele (which is the most frequent in the general population) with GD, but this effect could not be dissociated by the effect of the 49 A/G allele, indicating partial linkage disequilibrium (34). No evidence of association was found in a subsequent study, using both classical and family-based association analysis (35). Therefore this polymorphism does not appear to confer additional risk, over the one derived from the 49 A/G SNP.

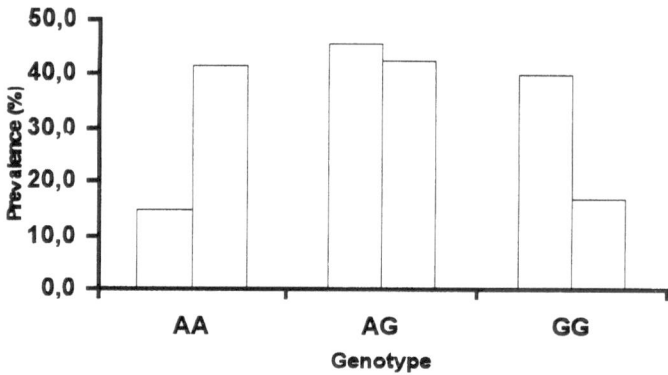

Figure 2. Distribution of the CTLA-4 49 A/G SNP alleles in the Japanese (left column) and Caucasian (right column) populations.

Linkage analyses with CTLA-4.

As summarized in the above paragraphs, CTLA-4 polymorphisms have shown to be associated with AITD significantly, but with small relative risks. This observation can be explained in two ways. The first possible explanation is that these polymorphisms only represent a small proportion of the whole genetic predisposition to the disease. Alternatively, the studied polymorphisms may in fact be mere markers, in only partial linkage disequilibrium with an unknown gene variation with an important genetic effect. In the latter situation not all affected carriers would also carry the associated allele and a relevant proportion of unaffected subjects would carry it, yielding small relative risks in both classical and family-based association studies. In contrast, in linkage analysis the co-segregation of alleles of polymorphic markers with the disease phenotype is analysed in families or siblings, allowing the detection of genetic determinants, independently of the single allele studied in each family. Linkage analysis is used to detect necessary genes with an important role in the genetic predisposition to complex heritable diseases (36). Linkage analysis is somewhat insensitive but when known candidate genes are studied, in a sufficiently large dataset, the choice of appropriate markers, very close to the target gene allows to increase greatly the power of the analysis. We have initially used this approach to study the role of CTLA-4 in the genetic predisposition to

114

AITD. We have employed the CTLA-4 3' microsatellite marker in a set of 48 multiplex families with AITD and analysed its co-segregation with the disease phenotype, defined as the presence or absence of clinical GD or HT. Our results excluded linkage of the CTLA-4 gene to the AITD phenotype, under a variety of inheritance models, suggesting that this gene may only have a small effect on the genetic predisposition to the clinically detectable diseases (37). At difference with our findings, another laboratory has reported linkage of AITD to the CTLA-4 locus, employing sib-pair analysis, a different type of linkage analysis that includes only affected subjects (38). In this report a non-parametric maximum LOD score of 3.46 for the CTLA-4 region was observed in a set of 77 AITD pairs, a relatively small sample for this kind of analyses. Recent data obtained in an extended dataset of AITD families by our group may help explain these discrepancies and are described in the following paragraphs.

One major component of the AITD phenotype is the presence of circulating anti-thyroglobulin, anti-thyroperoxidase or anti-TSH receptor antibodies (thyroid autoantibodies-Tab). It is however well known that TAb may also be found in subjects without clinical AITD (39). It has been also shown since many years that up to 50% of first degree relatives of AITD patients may have circulating TAb (40), suggesting a strong heritability of this trait. Moreover, segregation analyses have suggested a dominant mode of inheritance for TAb (41, 42). And indeed, in our collection of families, 34% of relatives of AITD patients had positive TAb tests, without overt AITD. We therefore decided to run a whole genome screen on this dataset, considering affected all patients with AITD (who of course also have positive TAb) and also their relatives with positive TAb tests and no overt AITD (17). Subjects in this latter group had been labelled as "non affected" in the previously reported analyses. The new dataset was composed of 56 AITD families, with 60 GD patients, 78 HT patients and 50 Tab positive relatives. By employing 387 microsatellite markers, spanning the whole genome, and applying classical two-point linkage analysis to each marker we observed a LOD score of 3.61 at the chromosomal region 2q33, containing the CTLA-4, CD28 and ICOS loci, with a dominant mode of inheritance and high penetrance (17). When analysing the new dataset for the AITD phenotype, no evidence of linkage to the AITD phenotype was observed, in keeping with our previous work (37). By fine mapping this region using densely spaced markers and applying multipoint linkage analysis, we restricted the maximum LOD score to a 4 cM region between markers D2S346 and D2S325. There was significant evidence of heterogeneity, indicating that in approximately 40% of our families there was linkage of the TAb positive phenotype to this locus. We then tested the prevalence of polymorphisms in the CTLA-4 and CD28 genes in the probands of linked families with ethnically matched healthy controls. The G allele of the 49 A/G CTLA-4 SNP was present in 84% of probands and 56% of controls. A novel CD28 SNP did not show any difference in its distribution between probands and controls. Because of the limited knowledge of the ICOS gene sequence, this gene was not tested (17).

Table 2. Available linkage studies of CTLA-4 and the AITD.

Reference	Phenotype	Dataset	Method	Max LOD score
Barbesino, 1998	GD	11 families	Classical linkage	-1.2
Barbesino, 1998	AITD	48 families	Classical linkage	-1.6
Vaidya, 1999	GD	71 sibpairs	Sibpair analysis	3.1
Vaidya, 1999	AITD	77 sibpairs	Sibpair analysis	3.4
Tomer, 2001	TAb	56 families	Classical linkage	3.6

How do these data compare with other studies (38) showing evidence of linkage of CTLA-4 with the AITD phenotype? (Table 2). One answer may reside in the different methods employed for detecting linkage. In their study, Vaydia and colleagues have used sibpair analysis (38). By this method, only affected sibpairs are studied. Since by definition most if not all AITD patients are also TAb positive, in the affected-only analysis testing for AITD is equivalent to testing the TAb phenotype. Hence, the observed positive linkage may be applied to both phenotypes. In contrast, classical linkage analysis draws segregation information not only from affected subjects, but also from their unaffected relatives, allowing the definition of different phenotypes in the same dataset. In summary, current evidence from linkage studies seems to indicate that region 2q33 contains a major determinant of the genetic susceptibility to development of TAb, as a distinct part of the AITD phenotype and that this major determinant is CTLA-4. However CTLA-4 is not responsible alone for the development of overt AITD. Indeed, we have shown in other studies, that other loci across the genome are linked to the GD, the HT and the AITD phenotype (43).

Functional studies.

Linkage analysis maps susceptibility loci for diseases, but cannot give any information on their structure or function. In contrast, association studies may indicate gene variations directly responsible for the disease being studied, although they may also simply indicate linkage disequilibrium with truly causative and still unknown gene variations in the same chromosomal region. In both cases, once a candidate gene or a candidate gene variation has been identified, functional studies are needed to verify its role in the pathogenesis of the target disease. Indirect evidence for an involvement of CTLA-4 in auto-immune diseases comes from animal studies. Indeed, mice lacking a functional CTLA-4 gene display a strikingly severe disease, characterized by massive lymphocytic infiltration of multiple organs and early mortality, although the characteristics of this disease have not been studied at the cellular level (8). Moreover, diabetes prone NOD mice show a reduced expression of CTLA-4 (44). While these studies show the importance of CTLA-4 in the physiology of tolerance, they still don't answer the question as to whether a deficiency of CTLA-4 signalling can explain autoimmune diseases in humans. Very recently preliminary studies have started to unravel the possible cellular and molecular mechanisms by which CTLA-4 gene variations may affect the immune re-sponse in humans. Kouki and colleagues (45) have reported that lymphocytes from CTLA-4 49 G/G carriers show a lower degree of CTLA-4-dependent T-cell inhibition, regardless of the presence of AITD. These encouraging data represent the first step in confirming important suggestions coming from for-mal genetic studies.

Conclusive remarks

Genetic studies suggest that CTLA-4 represents an emerging candidate as a susceptibility gene for the AITD. Recent evidence however, indicates that CTLA-4 is not sufficient alone for the predisposition to the full phenotype of AITD, but it may explain some components of the disease, such as the presence of circulating autoantibodies. Because the same alleles of CTLA-4 have been shown to increase the risk for other autoimmune diseases, CTLA-4 may be a predisposing factor for autoimmunity in general, while other genes, possibly in epistatic relationship to CTLA-4 may determine the kind of autoimmune disease each single carrier will develop. Part of this specificity may be conferred by HLA haplotypes, which confer antigen-specificity to the process of antigen presentation, but other important genes have been mapped by whole genome screens and await further characterization.

References

1. Dariavach P, Mattei MG, Golstein P, Lefranc MP (1988) Human Ig superfamily CTLA-4 gene: chromosomal localization and identity of protein sequence between murine and human CTLA-4 cytoplasmic domains. Eur J Immunol. 18:1901-5.
2. Balzano C, Buonavista N, Rouvier E, Golstein P (1992) CTLA-4 and CD28: similar proteins, neighbouring genes. Int J Cancer Suppl. 7:28-32.
3. Hutloff A, Dittrich AM, Beier KC, et al (1999) ICOS is an inducible T-cell co-stimulator structurally and functionally related to CD28. Nature. 397:263-6.
4. Lafage-Pochitaloff M, Costello R, Couez D, et al (1990) Human CD28 and CTLA-4 Ig superfamily genes are located on chromosome 2 at bands q33-q34. Immunogenetics. 31:198-201.
5. Beier KC, Hutloff A, Dittrich AM, et al (2000) Induction, binding specificity and function of human ICOS. Eur J Immunol. 30:3707-3717.
6. June CH, Bluestone JA, Nadler LM, Thompson CB (1994) The B7 and CD28 receptor families. Immunol Today. 15:321-31.
7. Oosterwegel MA, Greenwald RJ, Mandelbrot DA, Lorsbach RB, Sharpe AH (1999) CTLA-4 and T cell activation. Curr Opin Immunol. 11:294-300.
8. Waterhouse P, Penninger JM, Timms E, et al (1995) Lymphoproliferative disorders with early lethality in mice deficient in Ctla-4. Science. 270:985-8.
9. Polymeropoulos MH, Xiao H, Rath DS, Merril CR (1991) Dinucleotide repeat polymorphism at the human CTLA-4 gene. Nucleic Acids Res. 19:4018.
10. Yanagawa T, Hidaka Y, Guimaraes V, Soliman M, DeGroot LJ (1995) CTLA-4 gene polymorphism associated with Graves' disease in a Caucasian population. J Clin Endocrinol Metab. 80:41-5.

11. Sale MM, Akamizu T, Howard TD, et al (1997) Association of auto-immune thyroid disease with a microsatellite marker for the thyrotropin receptor gene and CTLA-4 in a Japanese population [In Process Citation]. Proc Assoc Am Physicians. 109:453-61.

12. Nistico L, Buzzetti R, Pritchard LE, et al (1996) The CTLA-4 gene region of chromosome 2q33 is linked to, and associated with, type 1 diabetes. Belgian Diabetes Registry. Hum Mol Genet. 5:1075-80.

13. Badenhoop K, Donner H, Braun J, Siegmund T, Rau H, Usadel KH (1996) Genetic markers in diagnosis and prediction of relapse in Graves' disease. Exp Clin Endocrinol Diabetes. 104:98-100.

14. Donner H, Rau H, Walfish PG, et al (1997) CTLA4 alanine-17 confers genetic susceptibility to Graves' disease and to type 1 diabetes mellitus. J Clin Endocrinol Metab. 82:143-6.

15. Heward JM, Allahabadia A, Armitage M, et al (1999) The development of Graves' disease and the CTLA-4 gene on chromosome 2q33. J Clin Endocrinol Metab. 84:2398-401.

16. Kotsa K, Watson PF, Weetman AP (1997) A CTLA-4 gene polymorphism is associated with both Graves disease and autoimmune hypothyroidism. Clin Endocrinol (Oxf). 46:551-554.

17. Tomer Y, Greenberg DA, Barbesino G, Concepcion E, Davies TF (2001) Ctla-4 and not cd28 is a susceptibility gene for thyroid autoantibody production. J Clin Endocrinol Metab. 86:1687-93.

18. Donner H, Braun J, Seidl C, et al (1997) Codon 17 polymorphism of the cytotoxic T lymphocyte antigen 4 gene in Hashimoto's thyroiditis and Addison's disease. J Clin Endocrinol Metab. 82:4130-2.

19. Waterman EA, Watson PF, Lazarus JH, Parkes AB, Darke C, Weetman AP (1998) A study of the association between a polymorphism in the CTLA-4 gene and postpartum thyroiditis. Clin Endocrinol (Oxf). 49:251-5.

20. Chen QY, Nadell D, Zhang XY, et al (2000) The human leukocyte antigen HLA DRB3*020/DQA1*0501 haplotype is associated with Graves' disease in African Americans. J Clin Endocrinol Metab. 85:1545-9.

21. Petrone A, Giorgi G, Mesturino CA, et al (2001) Association of DRB1*04-DQB1*0301 haplotype and lack of association of two polymorphic sites at CTLA-4 gene with Hashimoto's thyroiditis in an Italian population. Thyroid. 11:171-5.

22. Vaidya B, Imrie H, Perros P, et al (1999) Cytotoxic T lymphocyte antigen-4 (CTLA-4) gene polymorphism confers susceptibility to thyroid associated orbitopathy. Lancet. 354:743-4.

23. Buzzetti R, Nistico L, Signore A, Cascino I (1999) CTLA-4 and HLA gene susceptibility to thyroid-associated orbitopathy. Lancet. 354:1824.

24. Villanueva R, Inzerillo AM, Tomer Y, et al (2000) Limited genetic susceptibility to severe Graves' ophthalmopathy: no role for CTLA-4 but evidence for an environmental etiology. Thyroid. 10:791-8.

25. Bartalena L, Pinchera A, Marcocci C (2000) Management of Graves' ophthalmopathy: reality and perspectives. Endocr Rev. 21:168-99.

26. Agarwal K, Jones DE, Daly AK, et al (2000) CTLA-4 gene polymorphism confers susceptibility to primary biliary cirrhosis. J Hepatol. 32:538-41.

27. Agarwal K, Czaja AJ, Jones DE, Donaldson PT (2000) Cytotoxic T lymphocyte antigen-4 (CTLA-4) gene polymorphisms and susceptibility to type 1 autoimmune hepatitis. Hepatology. 31:49-53.

28. Awata T, Kurihara S, Iitaka M, et al (1998) Association of CTLA-4 gene A-G polymorphism (IDDM12 locus) with acute-onset and insulin-depleted IDDM as well as autoimmune thyroid disease (Graves' disease and Hashimoto's thyroiditis) in the Japanese population. Diabetes. 47:128-9.

29. Djilali-Saiah I, Schmitz J, Harfouch-Hammoud E, Mougenot JF, Bach JF, Caillat-Zucman S (1998) CTLA-4 gene polymorphism is associated with predisposition to coeliac disease. Gut. 43:187-9.

30. Fukazawa T, Yanagawa T, Kikuchi S, et al (1999) CTLA-4 gene polymorphism may modulate disease in Japanese multiple sclerosis patients. J Neurol Sci. 171:49-55.

31. Huang D, Giscombe R, Zhou Y, Lefvert AK (2000) Polymorphisms in CTLA-4 but not tumor necrosis factor-alpha or interleukin 1beta genes are associated with Wegener's granulomatosis. J Rheumatol. 27:397-401.

32. Ligers A, Xu C, Saarinen S, Hillert J, Olerup O (1999) The CTLA-4 gene is associated with multiple sclerosis. J Neuroimmunol. 97:182-90.

33. Deichmann K, Heinzmann A, Bruggenolte E, Forster J, Kuehr J (1996) An Mse I RFLP in the human CTLA4 promotor. Biochem Biophys Res Commun. 225:817-8.

34. Braun J, Donner H, Siegmund T, Walfish PG, Usadel KH, Badenhoop K (1998) CTLA-4 promoter variants in patients with Graves' disease and Hashimoto's thyroiditis. Tissue Antigens. 51:563-6.

35. Heward JM, Allahabadia A, Carr-Smith J, et al (1998) No evidence for allelic association of a human CTLA-4 promoter polymorphism with autoimmune thyroid disease in either population-based case-control or family-based studies. Clin Endocrinol (Oxf). 49:331-4.

36. Greenberg DA (1993) Linkage analysis of "necessary" loci versus "susceptibility" loci. Am J Hum Genet. 52:135-143.

37. Barbesino G, Tomer Y, Concepcion E, Davies TF, Greenberg DA (1998) Linkage analysis of candidate genes in autoimmune thyroid disease: 1. Selected immunoregulatory genes. International Consortium for the Genetics of Autoimmune Thyroid Disease. J Clin Endocrinol Metab. 83:1580-4.

38. Vaidya B, Imrie H, Perros P, et al (1999) The cytotoxic T lymphocyte antigen-4 is a major Graves' disease locus. Hum Mol Genet. 8:1195-9.

39. Mariotti S, Sansoni P, Barbesino G, et al (1992) Thyroid and other organ-specific autoantibodies in healthy centenarians. Lancet. 339:1506-1508.

40. Hall R, Owen SG, Smart GA (1960) Evidence for a genetic predisposition to formation of thyroid autoantibodies. Lancet. ii:187-188.

41. Phillips D, McLachlan S, Stephenson A, et al (1990) Autosomal dominant transmission of autoantibodies to thyroglobulin and thyroid peroxidase. J Clin Endocrinol Metab. 70:742-6.

42. Pauls DL, Zakarija M, McKenzie JM, Egeland JA (1993) Complex segregation analysis of antibodies to thyroid peroxidase in Old Order Amish families [see comments]. Am J Med Genet. 47:375-9.

43. Tomer Y, Barbesino G, Greenberg DA, Concepcion E, Davies TF (1999) Mapping the major susceptibility loci for familial Graves' and Hashimoto's diseases: evidence for genetic heterogeneity and gene interactions. J Clin Endocrinol Metab. 84:4656-64.

44. Colucci F, Bergman ML, Penha-Goncalves C, Cilio CM, Holmberg D (1997) Apoptosis resistance of nonobese diabetic peripheral lymphocytes linked to the Idd5 diabetes susceptibility region. Proc Natl Acad Sci U S A. 94:8670-4.

45. Kouki T, Sawai Y, Gardine CA, Fisfalen ME, Alegre ML, DeGroot LJ (2000) CTLA-4 gene polymorphism at position 49 in exon 1 reduces

the inhibitory function of CTLA-4 and contributes to the pathogenesis of Graves' disease. J Immunol. 165:6606-11.

Association of AITD with microsatellite markers for TSHR and CTLA-4 in Japanese patients

Takashi Akamizu M.D.
Department of Medicine and Clinical Science, Kyoto University Graduate School of Medicine, Kyoto 606-8507, Japan

Summary

We examined the genetic contribution of the thyrotropin receptor (TSHR) gene to autoimmune thyroid disease (AITD) in Japanese patients. We identified a dinucleotide repeat polymorphism near the *TSHR* gene which was mapped to an 8.6 cM interval between D14S74 and D14S55 on the long arm of human chromosome 14. TSHR-CA has been mapped to approximately 600kb of the TSHR gene using the radiation hybrid mapping. Initial studies with this marker, TSHR-CA, revealed a significant association between AITD and one specific allele (allele 1) of the microsatellite sequence in 81 unrelated Japanese AITD patients and 113 Japanese controls (Sale et al., Proc. Assoc. Am. Physicians, 109:453, 1997). In a second study, TSHR-CA and another TSHR microsatellite marker, TSHR-AT, which is located in intron 2 of TSHR gene (de Roux et al., Mol Cell Endocrinol, 117:253, 1996), were genotyped in a set of 349 unrelated Japanese AITD patients and 218 Japanese controls. The TSHR-AT marker showed an association in this Japanese AITD population with a significant increase in allele 5 (294 bp; $P < 0.05$) and a significant decrease in allele 7 (298 bp; $P < 0.05$). The association of allele 5 of TSHR-AT was also significant in hypothyroid patients (TBII+, $P < 0.01$; TBII-, $P < 0.05$), as was .the association of allele 7 of TSHR-AT ($P < 0.05$). Associations with TSHR-CA were observed in patients with Hashimoto's thyroiditis (HT) with respect to alleles 3 (179 bp; $P < 0.05$) and 5 (175 bp; $P < 0.05$) and with hypothyroid TBII- patients for allele 4 (177 bp; P < 0.05). (Akamizu et al. Thyroid, 10: 851, 2000).

The *cytotoxic T lymphocyte antigen-4 (CTLA-4)* gene was also genotyped in this expanded set of Japanese AITD patients and controls. Associations between AITD susceptibility and allele 2 (102 bp; P < 0.01) and allele 4 (106 bp; P < 0.01) were observed. These associations were also observed in patients with Graves' disease (GD) (allele 2, P < 0.01; allele 4, P < 0.01).

The presence of specific alleles of TSHR-CA, TSHR-AT, and CTLA-4 contribute a significant increase in risk of development of AITD. These findings suggest that alleles of the *TSHR* and *CTLA-4* genes, or genes near them, contribute to AITD susceptibility and set the stage for future studies on the interactions between these genes and AITD.

Key Words
autoimmune thyroid disease, Graves' disease, Hashimoto's thyroiditis, susceptible gene, thyrotropin receptor, CTLA-4, microsatellite marker, association study

1. Genetic contribution of the TSHR gene to AITD

1) TSHR polymorphisms

TSHR is one of the major thyroid specific antigens. Stimulating antibodies to TSHR have been found in patients with Graves' disease (GD), an autoimmune disorder characterized by hyperthyroidism, while TSHR blocking antibodies have been detected in some non-goitrous hypothyroid patients (1). Point mutations have been identified in putative ligand binding regions of the extracellular domain of the *TSHR* gene in patients with GD (2-4), and these mutations may produce autoantigens involved in pathogenesis of the disease. However, no consensus has been established concerning their association or linkage with GD or AITD (Table 1). For example, Cuddihy et al. (5) showed a significant association of P52T with AITD in females, but Watson et al. (6) did not find the association with GD. We did not observe the *TSHR* codon 52 (C_{52} to A_{52}) transition mutation in any Japanese AITD patients (7). We found a significant association between AITD in Japanese patients and one specific allele of the microsatellite sequence, TSHR-CA (7), while de Roux et al., did not find a significant linkage between GD in Welsh and English populations and any alleles of another microsatellite marker, TSHR-AT (8).

Table 1. Polymorphisms of TSH receptor genes

---

1. Polymorphisms of coding regions of TSH Receptor Gene
1) P52T
    Association with AITD in females (Ref. 5)
    Lack of association with Graves' disease (Ref. 6)
2) D727E - no association with Graves' disease (Ref. 7)
    1) D36H – no full study

2. Microsatellite markers within or near TSH receptor gene
1) TSHR-AT: intron 2
    No linkage with Graves' disease in Welsh and English (Ref. 8)
2) TSHR-CA: near TSHR gene
    Association with AITD in Japan (Ref. 7)

---

2) Association study of TSHR microsatellite markers in Japanese population

As mentioned above, our initial association studies using a TSHR-CA microsatellite marker closely linked to the TSHR gene showed a significant difference between the TSHR microsatellite allele frequency distribution in 81 unrelated Japanese AITD patients and 113 Japanese controls: a significant increase in one particular allele (allele 1) of the microsatellite sequence was observed (7). Although these results suggest that allele 1 of the TSHR microsatellite is associated with a susceptibility locus for AITD in Japanese patients, the association of allele 1 with GD was not significant when the AITD patients were separated on the basis of disease type. To extend the initial study, TSHR-CA and another TSHR microsatellite marker, TSHR-AT, which is located in intron 2 of TSHR gene (10), were genotyped in a set of 349 unrelated Japanese AITD patients and 218 Japanese controls. Association between TSHR microsatellite markers and AITD susceptibility was evaluated by the standard chi-square test and the Relative Predispostional Effect (RPE) method (11). The RPE approach starts with the calculation of expected frequencies across cases and controls for each pair of subject groups. The resulting chi-square statistic for each allele has a single degree of freedom (df). Rather than recalculating the expectations after each evaluation of significance, only the initially significant allele is "removed" from the table and the chi-square tests are recalculated.

Table 2 shows the results of the association analysis of TSHR-CA and -AT polymorphism alleles and AITD (12). Significant differences between the allele frequencies of cases and controls are reported on the basis of allele-specific tests of significance, using a c^2 statistic with 1 degree of freedom. For the TSHR-CA polymorphism, allele 3 (179 bp) was decreased ($P < 0.10$) in AITD cases versus controls. This decrease was significant for HT cases ($P < 0.05$) and nearly significant ($P < 0.10$) in hypothyroid TSH binding inhibitor immunoglobulin (TBII) -negative cases. Allele 4 (177 bp) was significantly increased ($P < 0.05$) in hypothyroid TBII-positive cases, while allele 5 (175 bp) was significantly increased ($P < 0.05$) in HT cases. For the TSHR-AT polymorphism, allele 5 (294 bp) was significantly increased ($P < 0.05$) in AITD cases, hypothyroid TBII-positive cases ($P < 0.01$) and hypothyroid TBII-negative cases ($P < 0.05$). Allele 7 (298 bp) was significantly decreased in AITD cases ($P < 0.05$) and in hypothyroid TBII-positive cases ($P < 0.05$). Allele 19 (326 bp) was significantly ($P < 0.05$) increased in HT cases and was nearly significantly increased in AITD cases ($P < 0.10$). The analyses of the data using the RPE approach showed similar findings (Table 3, Ref. 12).

The increased risk for developing AITD in individuals with specific susceptibility alleles of TSHR-CA and TSHR-AT was evaluated by calculating the odds ratios, (i.e., risk ratios), as shown in Table 4 (12). For the TSHR-AT polymorphism the most strongly associated allele 5 showed an increased risk of 1.8 fold, which was statistically significant ($P=0.006$; Table 4).

Table 2. Polymorphism allele frequencies of TSHR markers in Japanese AITD patients and controls

Allele	bp	Controls[a]	AITD[a,b]	GD[a,b]	HT[a,b]	Hypothyroidism[a,b] TBII(+)	TBII(-)
TSHR-CA		n=312	n=668	n=366	n=192	n=64	n=46
1	183	0.035	**0.058**	0.052	0.058	0.078	0.087
2	181	0.186	**0.220**	**0.242**	0.195	0.172	0.217
3	179	0.455	**0.380**	0.402	**0.333**	0.469	0.283
4	177	0.048	**0.060**	0.063	0.037	0.063	**0.130**
5	175	0.269	0.263	0.221	**0.370**	0.203	0.239
Pooled alleles[c]		0.006	0.018	0.019	0.011	0.016	0.043
TSHR-AT		n=348	n=698	n=372	n=212	n=66	n=48
5	294	0.095	**0.156**	**0.161**	0.104	**0.258**	**0.208**
6	296	0.319	0.274	0.290	0.245	0.303	0.229
7	298	0.365	**0.281**	0.282	0.325	**0.182**	0.208
8	300	0.080	0.069	0.056	0.080	0.091	0.083
9	302	0.014	0.014	0.005	**0.038**	0.000	0.000
15	318	0.014	0.019	0.019	0.014	0.015	0.042
16	320	0.017	**0.033**	0.030	0.028	0.045	0.063
17	322	0.026	0.023	0.030	0.009	0.030	0.021
18	324	0.023	0.020	0.016	0.028	0.000	0.042
19	326	0.014	**0.033**	**0.03**	**0.042**	0.015	0.021
Pooled alleles[d]		0.032	0.079	0.078	0.085	0.061	0.083

[a] n=total number of alleles

[b] frequencies in bold type are significantly different in patients compared to frequencies in the conrols

[c] Pooled alleles control frequencies <0.015

[d] Pooled alleles: control frequencies <0.014

Table 3. RPE analysis of allelic associations with AITD

Disorder	n (CG*)	allele (no)	(bp)	allele specific chi-square (1 df[a])	total chi-square (all alleles, k[b] df)	'+'=risk '-' '-'=protection
TSHR-CA						
AITD	668				6.92	
GD	366				6.98	
HT	192	3	179	4.31	10.05	-
Hypo TBII+	64				2.91	
Hypo TBII-	46	4	177	4.64	10.29	+
TSHR-AT						
AITD	698	5	294	6.43	19.34	+
GD	372	5	294	6.15	17.77	+
HT	212	19	326	4.15	13.14	+
Hypo TBII+	66	5	294	12.17	20.71	+
Hypo TBII-	48	5	294	5.01	16.14	+

[a]df: degrees of freedom
[b]k: the number of alleles of each marker
*: chromosomes genotyped

Table 4. Risks associated with AITD susceptibility alleles of TSHR

LOCUS		CASES	CONTROLS	OR[a]	95% CI[b]	P value
TSHR-CA						
	"alleles 1, 2 or 4"	226	84	**1.4**	1.0-1.9	**0.030**
	NOT "alleles 1, 2					
	or 4"	442	228			
TSHR-AT						
	"allele 5" 294bp	109	33	**1.8**	1.2-2.7	**0.006**
	NOT "allele 5"					
	294bp	589	315			

[a]Odds Ratio
[b]Confidence Interval

2. Genetic contribution of the CTLA-4 gene to AITD

1) CTLA-4 polymorphisms

CTLA-4 molecule is co-expressed with CD28 on activated T-cells and interacts with B7 on antigen-presenting cells to stimulate T-cell proliferation (13). Three polymorphisms have been used to explore an association between the AITD and CTLA-4 gene: an (AT)n repeat in the 3'-untranslated region of exon 4 (14), an A to G polymorphism in exon 1 (15), and a C to T polymorphism in the promoter (16) (Fig. 1). Previously, an association was observed between a microsatellite sequence in the CTLA-4 gene and susceptibility to GD in Caucasians (17, 18) and to HT in Caucasians (18), but only a borderline association in autoimmune hypothyroidism and subgroups of AITD was observed in our previous study (7). The second polymorphism in the *CTLA-4* gene, A/G SNP[49] demonstrated evidence of an association between susceptibility to GD in Caucasians (19), Hong Kong Chinese (20), and Japanese Graves' patients (21). The third polymorphism, the SNP in the promoter, was associated with GD in Koreans (22).

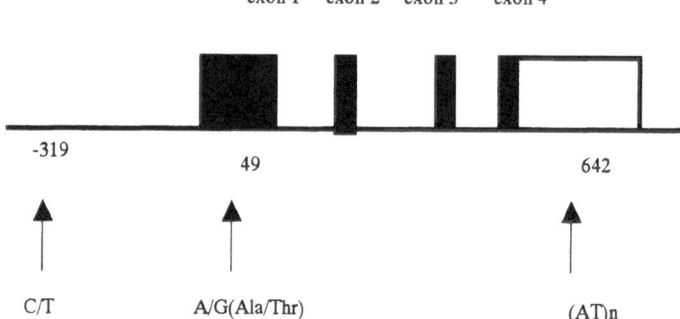

Chromosome 2q33

exon 1   exon 2   exon 3   exon 4

-319

49

642

C/T

A/G(Ala/Thr)

(AT)n

Fig. 1 Polymorphisms of human CTLA-4 gene. Ala/Thr:
alanine/threonine

2) Association study of CTLA-4 microsatellite marker in Japanese population

The CTLA-4 gene was also genotyped in this expanded set of Japanese AITD patients and controls. The CTLA-4 polymorphism, allele 2 (102 bp) was significantly increased in AITD cases (P < 0.01), GD cases (P < 0.01) and nearly significantly increased in HT cases (P < 0.10) (Table 5, 6, Ref. 12). Allele 4 (106 bp) was significantly decreased for AITD cases (P < 0.01), GD cases (P < 0.01) and nearly significantly decreased for HT cases (P < 0.10) and for hypothyroid TBII-positive cases (P < 0.10). The results with allele 4 suggested a protective effect on susceptibility to AITD, although it is difficult to know whether, when one allele enhances, decreased frequency of another allele means protective. This is the first report of such protective effect in CTLA-4 and is intriguing in terms of the function of the molecule. CTLA-4 is thought to functionally cooperate with CD28 on activated T lymphocytes (23), but it may have a protective/negative role in autoimmune diseases in contrast to CD28 (24, 25). Furthermore, CTLA-4 and CD28 may differentially activate the TH1/Th2 developmental pathways and affect the development of autoimmune diseases (26, 27).

The increased risk for developing AITD in individuals with specific susceptibility alleles of CTLA-4 was also evaluated by calculating the odds ratios as shown in Table 7. The major RPE associated allele (allele 2, 102bp) contributed significant increased risks (OR = 1.8). Consistent with the observed decrease of the frequency of allele 4 (106 bp) in AITD patients compared to controls, allele 4 is associated with a significantly reduced risk of 0.5, which is statistically significant (P= 0.0008).

Table 5. Polymorphism allele frequencies of CTLA-4 marker in Japanese AITD patients and controls

Allele		bp					Hypothyroidism	
			Controls	AITD	GD	HT	TBII(+)	TBII(-)
CTLA-4 AT								
			n=340	n=624	n=358	n=180	n=50	n=36
	1	88	0.306	0.253	0.239	0.241	0.380	0.278
	2	102	0.141	**0.224**	**0.239**	0.213	0.160	0.222
	3	104	0.215	**0.277**	**0.277**	0.278	0.300	0.250
	4	106	0.156	**0.085**	**0.086**	0.096	0.060	0.056
	5	108	0.085	0.077	0.067	0.079	0.100	0.139
	6	118	0.015	0.018	0.014	0.022	0.000	0.000
	7	122	0.026	0.013	0.011	0.017	0.000	0.028
Pooled alleles[e]			0.056	0.056	0.064	0.062	0.000	0.028

[e] Pooled alleles of 80, 82, 94, 100, 110, 112, 114, 116, 120, 124, 126, 128, 130bp (control frequencies <0.015).

frequencies in bold type are significantly different in patients compared to frequencies in the controls

Table 6. Predispositional Effect (RPE) analysis of allelic associations with AITD

Disorder	n (chromo-somes geno-typed)	allele (no)	allele (bp)	allele specific chi-square (1 df[a])	total chi-square (all alleles, [b]k df)	effect '+'=risk '-' =protection
CTLA-4						
AITD all	624	4	106	10.87	26.91	-
		2	102	7.80	16.04	+
GD	358	2	102	8.91	21.62	+
HT	180				11.58	
Hypo TBII+	50		d		8.13	
Hypo TBII-	36				5.54	

[a]df: degrees of freedom

[b]k: the number of alleles of each marker

Table 7. Risks associated with AITD susceptibility alleles of CTLA-4

LOCUS		CASES	CONT-ROLS	OR[a]	95% CI[b]	P value
CTLA-4-AT						
	"allele 2" 102bp	140	48	**1.8**	1.2 -2.5	**0.002**
	NOT "allele 2" 102bp	484	292			
	"allele 4" 106 bp	53	53	**0.5**	0.3 -0.8	**0.0008**
	NOT "allele 4" 106 bp	571	287			

[a]Odds Ratio

[b]Confidence Interval

3. Interactions between the TSHR-AT and CTLA-4 alleles associated with AITD

With evidence that alleles at multiple loci are associated with AITD or subgroups of AITD, possible interactions between these alleles were evaluated using 2X2 contingency tables to analyze the interactions. Odds ratios for different combinations of alleles of TSHR-CA, TSHR-AT, and CTLA4 were calculated, and their potential contributions to AITD susceptibility were assessed (Table 8, Ref. 12). Both χ^2 and Fisher Exact tests were carried out to evaluate the significance of these effects. When the two loci that seemed to contribute greater risk, TSHR-AT allele 5 and CTLA-4 allele 2, were evaluated together, it was interesting to observe that a combination of the two alleles did not appear to be associated with any increased risk for AITD (odds ratios approaching 1). This suggests that the TSHR-AT and CTLA-4 loci may be independent, rather than interacting, risk factors for AITD susceptibility. These interactions will need to be reevaluated with a larger dataset in order to fully evaluate their significance.

Table 8. Interaction Analysis:
CTLA4 102bp allele x TSHR-AT 294bp allele analysis

LOCUS		CASES	CONT-ROLS	OR[a]	95% CI[b]	P value
TSHR-AT allele 5						
	# with CTLA4 102 bp	37	11	1.0	0.45-2.0	0.92
	# without CTLA4 102 bp	151	43			
CTLA4 allele 102						
	# with TSHR-AT allele 5	37	11	0.9	0.44-1.9	0.81
	# without TSHR-AT allele 5	225	61			

[a]Odds Ratio
[b]Confidence Interval

Conclusion

We found significant associations of AITD and GD with microsatellite markers for the TSHR gene and CTLA-4 in a Japanese population. These findings suggest that alleles of the TSHR and CTLA-4 genes, or genes near them, contribute to AITD susceptibility, and set the stage for future studies on the interactions between these genes and AITD.

References

1. Akamizu T, Kohn LD, Mori T (1995) Molecular studies on thyrotropin (TSH) receptor and anti-TSH receptor antibodies. Endocrine J 42:617-627
2. Heldin N-E, Gustavsson B, Westermark K, Westermark B (1991) A somatic point mutation in a putative ligand binding domain of the TSH receptor in a patient with autoimmune hyperthyroidism. J. Clin. Endocrinol. Metab. 73: 1374-1376
3. Bohr URM, Behr M, Loos U (1993) A heritable point mutation in an extracellular domain of the TSH receptor involved in the interaction with Graves' immunoglobulins. Biochim Biophys Acta 1216: 504-505.
4. Bahn RS, Dutton CM, Heufelder AE, Sarkar GA(1994) genomic point mutation in the extracellular domain of the thyrotropin receptor in patients with Graves' ophthalmopathy. J. Clin. Endocrinol. Metab. 78: 256-260.
5. Cuddihy R.M., Dutton C.M. and Bahn R.S. A (1995) polymorphism in the extracellular domain of the thyrotropin receptor is highly associated with autoimmune thyroid disease in females. Thyroid 5: 89-95.
6. Watson P.F., French A., Pickerill A.P., McIntosh R.S. and Weetman A.P (1995) Lack of association between a polymorphism in the coding region of the thyrotropin receptor gene and Graves' disease. J. Clin Endocrinol. Metab. 80: 1032-1035.
7. Sale MM, Akamizu T, Howard TD, Yokota T, Nakao K, Mori T, Iwasaki H, Rich SS, Jennings-Gee JE, Yamada M, Bowden DW (1997) Association of autoimmune thyroid disease with a microsatellite marker for the thyrotropin receptor gene and CTLA-4 in a Japanese population. Proc Assoc Amer Physician. 109:453-461.
8. de Roux N, Shields DC, Misrahi M, Ratanachaiyavong S, McGregor AM, Milgrom E (1996) Analysis of the thyrotropin receptor as a candidate gene in familial Graves' disease. J Clin Endocrinol Metab. 81: 3483-3486.
9. Muhlberg T, Herrmann K, Joba W, Kirchberger M, Heberling HJ, Heufelder AE (2000) Lack of association of nonautoimmune hyperfunctioning thyroid disorders and a germline polymorphism of codon 727 of the human thyrotropin receptor in a European Caucasian population. J Clin Endocrinol Metab. 85:2640-3.

10. de Roux N, Misrahi M, Chatelain N, Gross B, Milgrom E (1996) Microsatellites and PCR primers for genetic studies and genomic sequencing of the human TSH receptor gene. Mol Cell Endocrinol 117: 253-256.

11. Payami H, Joe S, Farid NR, Stenszky V, Chan S., Yeo PPB, Cheah JS Thomson G (1989) Relative predispositional effects (RPEs) of marker alleles with disease: HLA-DR alleles and Graves' Disease. Am J Hum Genet. 45: 541-546.

12. Akamizu T, Sale MM, Rich SS, Hiratani H, Yoshimura Noh J, Saijo M, Moriyama K, Miyamoto Y, Saito Y, Nakao K, Bowden DW (2000) Association of autoimmune thyroid disease with microsatellite markers for the thyrotropin receptor gene and CTLA-4 in Japanese patients. Thyroid, 10: 851-858.

13. Linsley PS, Brady W, Urnes M, Grosmaire LS, Damle NK, Ledbetter JA (1991) CTLA-4 is a second receptor for the B-cell activation antigen B7/BB-1. J Exp Med. 174:561-569.

14. Polymeropoulos MH, Xiao H, Rath DS, Merril CR (1991) Dinucleotide repeat polymorphism at the human CTLA4 gene. Nucleic Acids Res. 19:4018.

15. Harper K, Balzano C, Rouvier E, Mattei MG, Luciani MF, Golstein P (1991) CTLA-4 and CD28 activated lymphocyte molecules are closely related in both mouse and human as to sequence, message expression, gene structure, and chromosomal location. J Immunol. 147:1037-44.

16. Deichmann K, Heinzmann A, Bruggenolte E, Forster J, Kuehr J (1996) An Mse I RFLP in the human CTLA4 promotor. Biochem Biophys Res Commun. 225:817-8.

17. Yanagawa T., Hidaka Y., Guimaraes V., Soliman M. and DeGroot L.J (1995) CTLA-4 gene polymorphism associated with Graves' disease in a Caucasian population. J. Clin. Endocrinol. Metab. 80: 41-45.

18. Kotsa K, Watson F, Weetman AP (1997) A CTLA-4 gene polymorphism is associated with both Graves' disease and autoimmune hypothyroidism. Clin Endocrinol (Oxf) 46: 551-554.

19. Donner H., Rau H., Walfish P.G., Braun J., Siegmund T., Finke R., Herwig J, Usadel K.H. and Badenhoop K (1997) CTLA4 alanine-17 confers genetic susceptibility to Graves' Disease and to Type 1 Diabetes Mellitus. J. Clin. Endocrinol. Metab. 82: 143-146.

20. Nisticò L, Buzzetti R, Pritchard LE, Van der Auwera B, Giovannini C, Bosi E, Martinez Larrad MT, Serrano Rios M, Chow CC, Cockram

CS, Jacobs K, Mijovic C, Bain SC, Barnett AH, Vandewalle CL, Schuit F, Gorus FK, Belgian Diabetes Registry, Tosi R, Pozzilli P and Todd JA (1996) The CTLA-4 gene region of chromosome 2q33 is linked to, and associated with, type 1 diabetes. Hum Mol Genet. 5: 1075-1080.

21. Yanagawa T, Taniyama M, Enomoto S, Gomi,K, Maruyama H, Ban Y, Saruta T (1997) CTLA-4 gene polymorphism confers susceptibility to Graves' disease in Japanese. Thyroid. 7: 843-846.

22. Park YJ, Chung HK, Park DJ, Kim WB, Kim SW, Koh JJ, Cho BY (2000) Polymorphism in the promoter and exon 1 of the cytotoxic T lymphocyte antigen-4 gene associated with autoimmune thyroid disease in Koreans. Thyroid. 10:453-9.

23. Linsley PS, Greene JL, Tan P, Bradshaw-J; Ledbetter JA, Anasetti C, Damle NK (1992) Coexpression and functional cooperation of CTLA-4 and CD28 on activated T lymphocytes. J Exp Med. 176:1595-1604

24. Walunas TL, Bakker CY, Bluestone JA (1996) CTLA-4 ligation blocks CD28-dependent T cell activation. J Exp Med. 183:2541-2550.

25. Kearney ER, Walunas TL, Karr PA, Morton PA, Loh DY, Bluestone JA, Jenkins MK (1995) Antigen-dependent clonal expansion of a trace population of antigen-specific CD4+ T cells in vivo is dependent on CD28 costimulation and inhibited by CTLA-4. J Immunol. 155:1032-1036.

26. Kuchroo VK, Das MP, Brown JA, Ranger AM, Zamvil SS, Sobel RA, Weiner HL, Nabavi N, Glimcher LH (1995) B7-1 and B7-2 costimulatory molecules activate differentially the Th1/Th2 developmental pathways: application to autoimmune disease therapy. Cell. 80:707-718.

27. Lenschow DJ, Ho SC, Sattar H, Rhee L, Gray G, Nabavi N, Herold KC, Bluestone JA (1995) Differential effects of anti-B7-1 and anti-B7-2 monoclonal antibody treatment on the development of diabetes in the nonobese diabetic mouse. J Exp Med. 181:1145-1155.

Part 2

Familial Thyroid Cancers

Familial Non Medullary Thyroid Cancer

Orlo H Clark, M.D.
Department of Surgery, University of California San Francisco Medical
School UCSF/Mt Zion Medical Center, San Francisco, CA, USA

Key Words
familial thyroid cancer, familial medullary thyroid cancer, Familial non medullary thyroid cancer, FNMTC, Hurthle cell, papillary thyroid cancer, multiple endocrine neoplasia, MEN, RET, PTC, Cowden's syndrome, familial polyposis.

When one thinks about patients with familial thyroid cancer, one usually considers familial medullary thyroid cancer or perhaps familial thyroid cancers associated with familial polyposis or Cowden's syndromes. However, there have been an increasing number of articles regarding patients with FNMTC in the past few years [1-16]. Familial non medullary thyroid cancer (FNMTC) without any other associated syndrome, however, accounts for about 5% of patients with thyroid cancer of follicular cell origin (prevalence ranges between 3.5 and 6.2%) [1, 17, 18]. FNMTC has been defined as families with two or more first degree relatives having cancer papillary or Hurthle cell thyroid. In patients with three or more members with thyroid cancer there appears to be an autosomal dominant type of inheritance with incomplete penetrance and 99.9% of these patients have familial disease [2]. Patients with FNMTC also are more likely to have other thyroid pathology including multinodular goiter as well as other non thyroid cancers [3]. When two members of a family have thyroid cancer some will have a susceptibility gene for thyroid cancer; the others may have sporadic non familial tumors [2].

During the past ten years there have been dramatic advances in the earlier diagnosis of familial diseases by genetic testing rather than by physiologic testing or by physical examination. For example, about 98% of the genes responsible for familial medullary thyroid carcinoma (FMTC) including multiple endocrine neoplasia 2A – 2B have been identified on chromosome 10 [18-22]. It is generally agreed that all patients with MTC should be screened for RET point mutations because de novo mutations occur in about 10% of patients with FMTC and MEN2A, and in about 50% of those with MEN2B [23, 24]. Since there is nearly 100% penetrance of the MTC, screening for a germ line. RET mutation should be done in MEN2A and FMTC before age six and in MEN2B suspected patients at 1 year of age. Prophylactic surgical treatment, that is total thyroidectomy with or without central neck dissection depending on whether medullary thyroid cancer is present, should be done in all patients with a RET mutation that has been confirmed once (done twice) in patients from families with familial MTC. [21}

Our policy is to recommend basal and stimulated calcitonin (CT) tests and ultrasound examination of the neck including thyroid and adjacent nodes in patients who are RET positive [21]. When the CT levels are increased or the ultrasound shows any lesions in the thyroid gland a total thyroidectomy and bilateral central neck dissection is recommended. The parathyroid glands should be marked with clips, because about 20% of patients with MEN 2A will develop primary hyperparathyroidism. If central neck nodes are positive or the primary tumor is larger than 1.5 cm an ipsilateral modified radical neck dissection should also be done. This procedure, however, is rarely necessary in young patients identified by RET testing. When the CT levels are low or normal and there are no nodules on ultrasound, a total thyroidectomy without prophylactic central neck dissection should be done, and the parathyroid glands preserved and marked with a clip as mentioned. [6] Although some authorities recommend waiting until the calcitonin levels increase in RET positive patients we believe that delaying treatment might allow the tumor to grow and metasize thus requiring more extensive surgery with an increased risk of complications and greater chance of persistent or recurrent MTC.

To date, genetic testing to document whether an individual of a family with familial papillary or Hurthle cell cancer without other syndromes has a specific germ line mutation is not available. Since about 5% of patients with papillary and Hurthle cell cancer have familial thyroid cancer without any other syndromes FNMT is more common than FMTC [3, 9, 17]. FNMTC also occurs more commonly in association with the rare syndromes of Cowden's syndrome [25, 26], familial polyposis [8,9], Carney's syndrome [27], Werner's syndromes in Japanese but not Caucasians [28, 29, 30] and probably in patients with familial hyperparathyroidism [31] and MEN1 [32]. FNMTC is rare in patients with follicular thyroid cancer but has been reported in patients with dyshormogenesis [33]. Familial papillary thyroid cancer has also currently been reported in families with papillary renal hyperplasia [7, 9].

Canzian et al [8] in 1998 identified a linkage site locus (thyroid cancer oxyophilia) (TCO gene) on chromosome 19p13.2 in a single French family with oxyophilia and trabecular thyroid cancers. We have confirmed this mutation in one of our families with familial Hurthle cell cancer [34]. Malcoff et al [7, 19] found a locus for familial PTC with papillary renal cell hyperplasia mapped to gene 1q21. This association is of interest since in contrast to most patients with thyroid cancer with TCO, and in patients with thyroid cancer and familial polyposis where there is a distant histological pattern respectively, patients with papillary thyroid cancer and renal cell hyperplasia have the same pattern as found in patients with sporadic papillary thyroid cancer. [7,9] Eng [18] also noted a possible association of clear cell renal cancer and familial papillary thyroid cancer "perhaps on gene 3p14 or 8q24". Two cases of occult papillary thyroid cancer were also identified in a large Canadian family with familial multinodular goiter. [35] This putative locus was mapped to chromosome 14q31, but the papillary cancers were thought to be incidental tumors in those patients [35].

All studies regarding genetic testing involve ethical issues and have potential serious psychological effects. Such investigations, therefore, require informed consent, clear discussion of the results of the testing and follow up counseling when necessary. It seems counter intuitive, however, not to identify individuals who have a susceptibility gene for FNMTC or other cancers when earlier treatment can improve outcome and decrease the risk of recurrent tumor or premature death from this tumor. Genetic testing also relieves the anxiety of having an increased risk of cancer in family members who are germ line negative for the susceptibility gene. However, there is still concern about potential problems such as being refused health insurance or the necessity of paying higher fees for health life insurance. Our own studies and others document that it appears to be cost effective to screen for familial diseases when currently available therapy is available that results in improved therapy because of earlier diagnosis [36, 37]. Genetic counselors must be members of the clinical and scientific research team to help counsel and advise patients with possible familial disease.

History

The familial occurrence of thyroid cancer was first noted in tumor in 1955 and also in kindreds with familial adenomatous polyposis in 1968 [38, 39]. Numerous reports have subsequently been published [25,26,38,39]. Most reported cases involve only two family members so that the one might question whether there is a true genetic predisposition or whether environmental factors are involved [2]. The current definition of FNMTC as briefly mentioned previously is a family having two first degree relatives with thyroid cancer without other syndromes such as Gardner's syndrome or Cowden's syndrome. Most studies suggest that benign thyroid disease is also more common in families with FNMTC [3]. Ron et al [40] found an odds ratio of five for patient with another family member with thyroid cancer, Goldger et al [41] using the Utah Population Database and Surveillance Epidemiology and End Results (SEER) data documented a 9 fold increase risk of thyroid cancer and an association with breast cancer (p < 0.001).

Our understanding of the genetic basis of autoimmune thyroid diseases advanced considerably during the past 5 years. The candidate gene approach and the genome-wide screening approach have both identified several chromosomal regions by linkage analysis in patients from families with Graves' disease including: MHC (6p21), CTLA-4 (2q23), GD2 (20p13), Xq21 (GD3), 14q31 (GD1), and Xp11 (NPL2.21) [42]. The reasons why different chromosomal regions have been identified by various investigators is not clear. Possible reasons for the findings include that a) some investigations only looked at a specific site, b) that the different chromosomal regions identified can possibly be explained by genetic heterogenicity between populations, c) by differences in familial structure or phenotypes, d) or by false positive linkage findings [43]. Although most thyroid cancers that occur in patients with Graves' disease are occult some coexisting thyroid cancers behave more aggressively [44]. Although this is attributed to stimulation of these cancers by thyroid stimulating antibodies or immunogloublins and other factors including genetic differences may be important.

Genetics and Environment

Studies by Burgess et al. [12] and our own investigations suggest that when three or more members of a family have papillary or Hurthle cell cancer, male to male transmission in successive generations, and horizontal presenta-

142

tion in siblings it supports an autosomal dominance mode of inheritance with incomplete expression [46]. When only two members in a family are involved a polygenetic mode of inheritance is more likely. A more thorough family history often identifies other family members with thyroid cancer.

Several reports suggest that thyroid cancer occurs more often in families with a clustering of other epithelial tumors including breast, skin and renal neoplasms [41, 42]. It has also been suggested from studies of families living near Chernobyl during the time of the nuclear disaster in 1986. Thus some families may be more susceptible to the oncogenic effects of radiation than others [46]. This is because in some families several children developed thyroid cancer whereas in others living in the same building no one developed thyroid cancer. Further investigations are necessary to confirm or refute this observation that there may be a genetic predisposition to develop cancer after radiation exposure in some individuals.

Previous studies have documented that the genes responsible for Cowden's disease (PTEN) and Gardner's disease or familial polyposis (APC) are not responsible for FNMTC [43, 48]. Cetta et al. [47, 48] have recently documented that most patients who have developed thyroid cancer who have familial polyposis not only have the germ line APC gene but also a RET/PTC somatic mutation in the thyroid. Other possible candidate genes for FNMTC because of their association with sporadic papillary thyroid cancer including TRK, RAS, C-MET have not been found to be responsible for FNMTC [8, 45]. As previously mentioned a linkage site mapped to chromosome 19p13.2 has been identified in a family with familial thyroid cancer with oxyophilia [8]. Another gene has been mapped to chromosome 1q21 in a family with familial papillary thyroid cancer and papillary renal neoplasms [7, 9]. Familial renal cell cancer and familial PTC may also occur in the same families [7,9]. Unfortunately these sites that have been identified by linkage analysis have not been found in other families with FNMTC and no other syndromes.

Pathology

The histologic finding relating to FNMTC seems to be unique in some families. Individuals with the TCO linkage site have a relatively characteristic histologic pattern with trabecular and oncocytic neoplasms [13]. Patients with papillary thyroid cancers and familial polyposis also have a distinct architecture and primarily occur in women [15, 16]. An experienced pathologist can make or at least suggest that the patient with this particular histological pattern should be screened for FNMTC. In contrast as previously mentioned papillary thyroid cancers associated with papillary renal neoplasia appear to be histologically similar to other papillary thyroid cancers without, at least obvious, histologic differences [7, 9].

Management

For patients presenting with a thyroid nodule or with documented papillary thyroid cancer or a Hurthle cell neoplasm by fine needle aspiration biopsy pathology warrants questions about other family members with thyroid cancer, other thyroid disorders and other tumors especially of the breast, kidney and colon. The documentation of a family history of these disorders increases the risk that other family members may be more susceptible or more at risk for thyroid cancer. A history of exposure to low dose or moderate dose therapeutic radiation is also important since it appears to increase the risk of not only thyroid cancer but also of parathyroid tumors, breast cancer and salivary gland tumors [49]. Earlier diagnosis and treatment results in improved outcome because the tumors are smaller and less invasive. As previously mentioned a history of irradiation does not exclude a familial predisposition to thyroid cancer and patients with FNMTC may be more susceptible to the oncogenic effects of radiation. As previously mentioned, a strong family history of benign thyroid disorders as well as one or more patients with thyroid helps to support the diagnosis of FNMTC.

The question of how to manage an individual in a family with other members who have familial papillary thyroid cancer or Hurthle cell cancer is most important. Certainly patients with thyroid nodules who have a family history of thyroid cancer are at high risk of having thyroid cancer. We consider these patients similar to patients with sporadic thyroid tumors and a history of exposure to low dose therapeutic irradiation. Numerous reports, including our own investigations, document that 40% of such patients have thyroid cancer in their thyroid glands [50, 51]. The index nodule is thyroid cancer 60% of the time when cancer is present in the thyroid gland but the presence of any thyroid nodule in a patient with a history of exposure to low dose therapeutic radiation must also be considered a harbinger of malignancy since 40% of the time thyroid cancer is situated elsewhere within the thyroid gland than in the thyroid nodule [50, 51].

Patients with thyroid nodules and other family members with thyroid cancer also have a marked increased risk of thyroid cancer and like patients with a history of radiation the cancers are more likely to be present in the presence of benign thyroid nodules [37, 45]. Thyroid cancer is also more likely to be multifocal in these patients. [37,45] We have previously reported that although the results of FNA cytology in family members of patients with FNMTC are not as accurate as in patients with presumed sporadic tumors, FNA biopsy still provides useful information [14].

Because of our own experiences and that reported by others, we recommend the same approach for patients in families with FNMTC that we do for patients with thyroid nodules and a history of radiation exposure that is total thyroidectomy with removal of regional lymphadenopathy when this operation can be done safely. We and others have reported that total thyroidectomy can be done with a complication rate of 1% or lower [52]. Among our patients with FNMTC we have had one patient with transient vocal cord palsy and no cases of hypoparathyroidism [45].

For individuals in families with two or more other members with papillary or Hurthle cell thyroid cancer and a normal thyroid gland to palpation we recommend a baseline ultrasound examination, to document whether there are any thyroid nodules present. If occult nodules are present they can be observed with a repeat ultrasound examination in six months and then yearly to be sure they are not growing, or they can be biopsied by FNA under ultrasound guidance. Although occult thyroid cancers are usually of little clinical significance this may not be true for patients with FNMTC. Lupoli et al. [53] reported that occult thyroid cancers in patients with FNMTC are more aggressive and may be lethal. Other studies by Osaki et al. [54], Grossman et al. [3], Takami et al. [55] have supported this conclusion although a study by Loh et al. [56] using metanalysis failed to support this conclusion. Alsanea and our group [45] therefore did a carefully controlled case study that strongly documented that familial papillary and Hurthle cell cancers are more likely to recur and to behave in a more aggressive manner.

Several groups continue to try to identify the genes responsible for the majority of families with FNMTC by linkage analysis, sib pair analysis and by the use of other investigations. Such studies are relatively expensive, but we believe are necessary if we are to improve the care of patients with FNMTC. The association of papillary thyroid cancer with breast and renal neoplasms may also provide new information about the etiology and growth of tumors in these patients.

References

1. Leprat F, Bonichon F, Guyot M, et al (1990) Familial non-medullary thyroid carcinoma: pathology review in 27 affected cases from 13 French families. Clin Endocrinol 50:589-594.
2. Charkes ND (1998) On the prevalence of familial nonmedullary thyroid cancer [letter]. Thyroid 8:857-8.
3. Grossman RF, Tu SH, Duh QY et al (1995) Familial nonmedullary thyroid cancer. An emerging entity that warrants aggressive treatment [see comments]. Arch Surg 130:892-7; discussion, 898-899.
4. Lupoli G, Vitale G, Caraglia M, et al (1999) Familial papillary thyroid microcarcinoma: a new clinical entity [see comments]. Arch Surg 353:637-639.
5. Burgess JR, Duffield A, Wilkinson SJ, et al (1997) Two families with an autosomal dominant inheritance pattern for papillary carcinoma of the thyroid. JCEM 82:345-348.
6. McKay JD, Williamson J, Lesueur F, et al (1999) At least three genes account for familial papillary thyroid carcinoma: TCO and MNG1 excluded as susceptibility loci from a large Tasmanian family. Eur J Endocrinol 141:122-125.
7. Malchoff CD, Sarfarazi M, Tendler B, et al (1999) Familial papillary thyroid carcinoma is genetically distinct from familial adenomatous polyposis coli. Thyroid 9:247-52.
8. Canzian F, Amati P, Harach HR, et al (1998) A gene predisposing to familial thyroid tumors with cell oxyphilia maps to chromosome 19p13.2. Am J Hum Genet 63:1743-48.
9. Malchoff CD, Sarfarazi M, Tendler B, Forouhar F, Whalen G, Joshi V, Arnold A, Malchoff DM (2000) Papillary thyroid carcinoma associated with papillary renal neoplasia: genetic linkage analysis of a distinct heritable tumor syndrome. JCEM 85:1758-64.
10. Lesueur F, Stark M, Tocco T, et al (1999) Genetic heterogeneity in familial nonmedullary thyroid carcinoma: exclusion of linkage to RET, MNG1, and TCO in 56 families. NMTC Consortium. JCEM 84:2157-2162.
11. Soravia C, Sugg SL, Berk T, et al (1999) Familial adenomatous polyposis-associated thyroid cancer: a clinical, pathological, and molecular genetics study. Am J Pathol 154:127-135.

12. Burgess JR, Dwyer T, McArdle K, et al (2000) The changing incidence and spectrum of thyroid carcinoma in Tasmania (1978-1998) during a transition from iodine sufficiency to iodine deficiency. JCEM 85:1513-1517.

13. Harach HR, Lesueur F, Amati P, et al (1999) Histology of familial thyroid tumours linked to a gene mapping to chromosome 19p13.2. J Pathol 189:387-93.

14. Vriens MR, Sabanci U, Epstein HD, et al (1999) Reliability of fine-needle aspiration in patients with familial nonmedullary thyroid cancer. Thyroid 9:1011-1016.

15. Perrier ND, van Heerden JA, Goellner JR, et al (1998) Thyroid cancer in patients with familial adenomatous polyposis. World J Surg 22:738-42; discussion, 743.

16. Harach HR, Soubeyran I, Brown A, et al (1999) Thyroid pathologic findings in patients with Cowden disease. Ann Diagnost Pathol 3:331-140.

17. Stoffen SS, Van Dyke DL, Bach JV, Szpunar W, Weiss L (1986) Familial papillary thyroid carcinoma of the thyroid. Am J Med Genet 25:775-782.

18. Eng C: Editorial (2000) Familial papillary thyroid cancer-many syndromes, too many genes? JCEM 85:1755-6.

19. 19. Phay JE, Moley JF, Lairmore TC (2000) Multiple endocrine neoplasias. Semin Surg Oncol 18:324-32.

20. 20. Heptulla RA, Schwartz RP, Bale AE, et al (1999) Familial medullary thyroid carcinoma: presymptomatic diagnosis and management in children. J Pediatric 135:327-331.

21. Kebebew E, Ituarte PH, Siperstein AE et al (2000) Medullary thyroid carcinoma: Clinical characteristics, treatment, prognostic factors, and a comparison of staging systems. Cancer 1139-1148.

22. Schuffenecker I; Virally-Monod M; Brohet R et al (1998) Risk and penetrance of primary hyperparathyroidism in multiple endocrine neoplasia type 2A families with mutations at codon 634 of the RET proto-oncogene. Groupe D'etude des Tumeurs a Calcitonine. JCEM, 83:487-91.

23. Carlson KM et 1 (1994) SIngle missense mutation in the tyrosine kinase catalytic domain of the RET rotooncogene is associated with MEN2B. Proc Natl Acad Sci USA, 91: 1579.

24.	Wells SA Jr; Franz C (2000) Medullary carcinoma of the thyroid gland. World Journal of Surgery, 24:952-6.
25.	Marsh DJ, Coulon V, Lunetta KL, et al (1998) Mutation spectrum and genotype-phenotype analyses in Cowden disease and Bannayan-Zonana syndrome, two hamartoma syndromes with germline PTEN mutation. Hum Mol Genet 7:507-515.
26.	Eng C (1999) The role of PTEN, a phosphatase gene, in inheritedand sporadic nonmedullary thyroid tumors. Recent Progr Horome Res 54:441-452; discussion, 453.
27.	Talpos GB (1997) In: Textbook of Endocrine Surgery. Non-Multiple Endocrine Neoplasia Endocrine Syndromes. (Clark OH and Duh QY eds). pp 635-641.
28.	Goto M, Miller RW, Ishikawa Y, et al (1996) Excess of rare cancers in Werner syndrome (adult progeria). Cancer Epidemiol Biomark Prevent 5:239-46.
29.	Ishikawa Y, Sugano H, Matsumoto T, et al (1999) Unusual features of thyroid carcinomas in Japanese patients with Werner syndrome and possible genotype-phenotype relations to cell type and race [see comments]. Cancer 85:1345-52.
30.	Nehlin JO, Skovgaard GL, Bohr VA (2000) The Werner syndrome. A model for the study of human aging. Ann N Y Acad Sci 908:167-179.
31.	Huang SM; Duh QY; Shaver J; Siperstein AE; Kraimps JL; Clark OH (1997) Familial hyperparathyroidism without multiple endocrine neoplasia. WJ Surg, 21:22-8.
32.	Kraimps JL, Duh QY, Demeure M, Clark OH (1992) Hyperparathyroidism in multiple endocrine neoplasia syndrome. Surgery 112: 1080-1085
33.	van de Graaf SA; Ris-Stalpers C; Veenboer GJ; Cammenga M (1999) A premature stopcodon in thyroglobulin messenger RNA results in familial goiter and moderate hypothyroidism. JCEM, 84:2537-42.
34.	Kraimps JL, Canzian, F, Jost C, Menet E et al (1999) Mapping of a gene disposing to familial thyroid tumors with cell oxyphilia to chromosome 19 and exclusion of JUN 8 as a candidate gene. Surgery 1188-94.
35.	Bignell GR, Cauzian F, Shayeghi M, et al (1997) Familial nontoxic multinodular goiter locus maps to chromosome 14q, but does not

account for familial nonmedullary thyroid cancer. Am J Hum Genet 61:1123-1130.

36. Dackiw A, Kuerer H, Clark OH. Current health care insurance policy for prophylactic thyroidectomy. (IAES 2001) Submitted World J Surg.

37. 37. Del bridge L, Robinson B(1998) Genetic and biochemical screening for endocrine disease: III. Cost and logistics. WJS 22: 1212-17.

38. Robinson D, Orr T (1955) Carcinoma of the thyroid and other diseases of the thyroid in identical twins. Arch Surg 70:923-28.

39. 39. Smith W (1968) Familial multiple polyposis: research tool for investigating the etiology of carcinoma of the colon? Dis Colon Rectum 11:17-31.

40. 40. Ron E, Kleinerman RA, LiVolsi VA, Fraumeni JF Jr (1991) Familial nonmedullary thyroid cancer. Oncology 48:309-311.

41. Goldgar DE, Easton DF, Cannon-Albright LA, Skolnick MH (1994) J National Cancer Institute 86:1600-8.

42. Imrie H, Vaidya B, Perros P, Kelley WF, Toft AD, Young ET, Kendall-Taylor P, Pearce SHS (2001) J Clin Endo & Metab 86:626-30.

43. Pearce SHS, Vaidya B, Imrie, et al (1999) Further evidence for a susceptibility locus on chromosome 20q13.11 in families with dominant transmission of Graves' disease. Am J Hum Genet 65:1462-5.

44. Filetti S; Belfiore A; Amir SM; Daniels GH; Ippolito O; Vigneri R; Ingbar SH (1988) The role of thyroid-stimulating antibodies of Graves' disease in differentiated thyroid cancer. NEJM, 318:753-9.

45. Alsanea O, Clark OH (2001) Familial thyroid cancer. Curr Opin Oncol 13:44-51.

46. Balter M (1996) Children become the first victims of fallout [news]. Science 272:357-60.

47. Cetta F; Gori M; Raffaelli N; Baldi C; Montalto G (1999) Comment on clinical and prognostic relevance of Ret-PTC activation in patients with papillary thyroid carcinoma [letter; comment]. JCEM 84:2257-8.

48. Cetta F; Olschwang S; Petracci M; Montalto G; Baldi C; Zuckermann M; Costantini RM; Fusco A (1998) Genetic alterations in

thyroid carcinoma associated with familial adenomatous polyposis: clinical implications and suggestions for early detection. W J Surgery 22:1231-6.

49. Perkel VS, Gail MH, Lubin J et al (1988) Radiation-induced thyroid neoplasms- evidence for familial susceptibility factors. JCEM 1316-22.

50. Miller AR; McBride WH; Hunt K; Economou JS (1994) Cytokine-mediated gene therapy for cancer. Annals of Surgical Oncology, 1(5):436-50.

51. Kikuchi S, Perrier N, Siperstein AE, et al. Evaluation of fine needle aspiration in patients with radiation induced thyroid neoplasm. Presented ATA 1999, October.

52. Grossman RF, Tu SH, Duh QY et al (1995) Familial non medullary thyroid cancer: An emerging entity that warrants aggressive treatment. Arch Surg 130z: 892-897.

53. Lupoli G, Vitale G, Caraglia M, et al (1999) Familial papillary thyroid microcarcinoma: a new clinical entity. Lancet 353:637-639.

54. Osaki D, Ito K, Kobayashi K, et al (1988) Familial occurrence of differentiated non medullary thyroid carcinoma. World J Surg 12:565-571

55. Takami H, Ozaki O Ito K (1996) Familial non medullary thyroid cancer: An emerging entity that warrants aggressive treatment. Arch Surg 131: 676.

56. Loh KC, Lo JC, Greenspan FS, Miller TR et al (1997) Familial papillary thyroid cancer: A case report. Ann Acad Med Singapore 26: 503-6.

Cowden Disease and the PTEN/MMAC1 Gene

[1]Bryan McIver, and [1,2]Norman L. Eberhardt
[1]Departments of Medicine and [2]Biochemistry & Molecular Biology, Mayo Clinic and Foundation, Rochester, Minnesota, USA

Key words
Cowden Disease, thyroid carcinoma, adenomatous goiter, follicular thyroid carcinoma, papillary thyroid carcinoma, chromosome 10q22-23, loss of heterozygosity, PTEN/MMAC1, Hürthle cell variant, phosphatase,

Cowden Disease: Clinical Phenotype and Pathophysiology.

Cowden Disease is a rare cancer predisposition syndrome, reported in 1963, and named after the first described patient[1]. She was a 20-year old woman with breast, skin and thyroid abnormalities, and with several developmental anomalies including *choanal atresia, pectus excavatum*, and mental retardation. In the initial case report, in addition to the developmental anomalies, the authors reported multiple papillomata of the lips and oropharynx, an unusual appearance of the tongue (scrotal tongue), breast hypertrophy, fibrocystic disease and recurrent breast ulceration, and an adenomatous goiter. The presence in the family of a *forme fruste* of the condition led them to suggest an inherited abnormality. Subsequently, 5 further similar cases were described[2], and the inheritance pattern was confirmed to be autosomal dominant. However, the phenotype, even within a family, is extremely variable, suggesting variable penetrance[3].

More than 200 families with Cowden Syndrome have now been described, and the International Cowden Consortium has developed diagnostic criteria, which are shown in Table 1. These criteria are dominated by the presence of characteristic skin lesions, which remain the most common feature

151

leading to the diagnosis. However, involvement of the breasts in female patients is almost universal, and thyroid involvement is also extremely common.

The dermatologic features including facial trichilemmomas, acral keratoses, and skin and mucosal papillomata, manifest in 100% of cases (see Table 1), and have a mean age at onset of 22 years (range 10-30)[4]. Figure 1 shows typical histologic features of a trichilemmoma from a patient with Cowden disease.

While Cowden syndrome is an inherited cancer predisposition syndrome, the majority of its features are in fact benign, with benign neoplasms affecting multiple organs including breast, thyroid, genitourinary tract, central nervous system, gastrointestinal tract and skeleton. The benign lesions that have been described are shown in Table 2. Malignant neoplasms are rather less common, but affect the breast in up to 30% of women, and the thyroid in 5-10% of cases[5]. All other reported malignancies have affected only a minority of patients, or represent occasional case reports.

Cowden Disease and the Thyroid

There is an almost 100% incidence of thyroid disease among patients with Cowden disease[6]. Most common are colloid or adenomatous goiters, there also seen frequently is hypothyroidism, subacute thyroiditis and occasional Graves' disease. In addition, thyroglossal duct cysts have been observed in these patients.

In the most extensive study yet published of thyroid findings in Cowden disease, Harach et al.[5] found multicentric follicular adenomas and adenomatous nodules in all 11 patients studied, ranging in size from microscopic to several centimeters. Forty-five percent of the adenomas were oxyphilic. Only 2 patients (18%) were shown to have follicular thyroid carcinoma (FTC), and these were both in patients over 40 years old. No other report exists specifically addressing thyroid findings in this condition. However, overall a 5-10% incidence of FTC has been described[4]. Interestingly, the original case report included a description of thyroid papillomatosis, but there are no other published case reports of patients with papillary thyroid carcinoma (PTC) in this condition. However, our own unpublished data from the Mayo Clinic have shown that PTC is in fact common in these patients (4/22 patients; 18.2%), while we have found no FTC in this group of patients. The reason for this discrepancy remains unknown, but could reflect differences between European and North American series, possibly due to differences in iodide intake. The outcomes of patients with Cowden disease treated for thyroid carcinoma remain unknown, and life expectancy is limited by breast carcinoma in females or other malignancies in men. No case reports have been published of Cowden patients dying of thyroid carcinoma. It seems likely that differentiated thyroid carcinoma arising in the context of Cowden disease behaves in the usual relatively indolent fashion and carries an excellent prognosis. However, multicentric disease is a possibility, which may justify a more aggressive initial therapeutic strategy[7].

Identification of the Cowden Gene

The chromosomal locus of the Cowden gene was identified in 1996 by Nelen et al.[8], who studied 12 families with the disease using a genome wide screening of 10 microsatellite markers per chromosome arm. They identified significant linkage with marker D10S573, mapped to chromosome 10q22-23, with a maximum LOD score of 8.92. The same region had already been identified as a site for frequent loss of heterozygosity (LOH) in multiple advanced carcinomas and was the target of investigation as a possible tumor suppressor gene locus. The putative tumor suppressor gene was identified in 1997 by two groups working independently and was named PTEN (phosphatase and tensin homologue deleted from chromosome 10)[9] and MMAC1 (mutated in multiple advanced cancers)[10]. High rates of LOH and homozygous deletions were identified by these groups in breast cancer, glioblastoma and other transformed cell lines. Confirmation that this putative tumor suppressor gene was also the gene responsible for Cowden disease came the same year with the finding of germ-line mutations of the PTEN/MMAC1 in 4/5 Cowden disease kindreds, and 19/29 unrelated cases[11,12]. Subsequent studies demonstrated that germ-line mutations of PTEN/MMAC1 are associated with three overlapping autosomal dominant disorders[13]. Cowden disease (CD), Bannayan-Zonana syndrome (BZS) and Lhermitte-Duclos disease (LDD). While BZS and LDD share some of the phenotypic features of CD, there are unique features to each of these conditions. The predominant phenotype of CD is skin hamartomas, although hamartomas are also found in breast, thyroid, endometrium, gastrointestinal tract and the central nervous system. The BZS phenotypes are very similar to CD with the exception of absence of hamartomas and epilepsy in the central nervous system, absence of benign tumors in breast heart/lung and bones, and lack of malignant breast, gastrointestinal and cutaneous tumors. Lhermitte-Duclos disease is characterized by a unique central nervous system disorder, cerebellar dysplastic gangliocytoma, but also includes many of the features of CD. While PTEN/MMAC1 mutations have been associated with each of this diseases, the determinants of the unique phenotypes remain to be elucidated.

In addition to heterozygous germ-line mutations the tumors of patients with Cowden disease exhibit reduced PTEN/MMAC1 mRNA expression at least in colonic polyps. This arises from deletion of the wild-type allele in some cases, but non-deletional mechanisms may also be important and hypermethylation of the wild-type allele has been reported[14].

PTEN/MMAC1 mutations have also been implicated in a minority of sporadic thyroid carcinoma. Frequent LOH is seen between 10q21 and 10q26, spanning the PTEN/MMAC1 locus, and this led to detailed mapping and mutation screening in sporadic thyroid cancers[15]. However, in a study of 17 FTC no mutations were identified with a single heterozygous mutation seen in 1/39 PTC. Nevertheless, low expression levels of PTEN/MMAC1 mRNA and protein have been observed in FTC[16], while mutations in Hürthle cell variant (oxyphilic) FTC may be more frequent, having been detected in 30% of this tumor type (McIver et al., unpublished data). All of these mutations were heterozygous, and no LOH was identified within the PTEN/MMAC1 locus in these tumors, but despite this, both PTEN/MMAC1 mRNA and protein expression were reduced, implicating this gene in the development or progression of the disease, and suggesting a non-deletional mechanism(s) of inactivation. These findings are discussed in more detail below.

Structure and Function of the PTEN/MMAC1 Gene

The predicted PTEN/MMAC1 protein product has the HCXXGXXR motif in its N-terminus that represents the canonical signature of protein tyrosine phosphatase and dual specificity protein phosphatase active sites. That PTEN/MMAC1 is a dual specificity phosphatase has been concluded from studies demonstrating that it can dephosphorylate highly acidic phosphorylated peptides containing tyrosine, serine or threonine[17]. Outside of the phosphatase domain there is very little homology to any of the known protein tyrosine phosphatase families. Instead the N-terminal region of PTEN/MMAC1 contains a domain with extensive homology to tensin and auxilin[10,18]. Tensin is a protein that interacts with actin filaments at focal adhesions, suggesting that PTEN/MMAC1 may suppress tumor cell growth by antagonizing protein tyrosine kinases and may regulate tumor cell invasion through interactions at focal adhesions. Support for this hypothesis come from data showing that confocal adhesion kinase (p125[FAK]) is an *in vitro* substrate for PTEN/MMAC1[19]. Auxilin is a brain-specific DnaJ homolog that is required for the chaperone Hsc70 to dissociate clathrin from bovine brain clathrin-coated vesicles[20]. Accordingly, PTEN/MMAC1 might conceivably be involved in membrane remodeling events that require exocytosis, including receptor recycling and down-regulation. The function of the C-terminal domain is not clear. This region includes a C2 lipid binding domain, which may be involved in binding phospholipid membranes[21], and several C-terminal phosphorylation sites that have been identified to be implicated in PTEN/MMAC1 stabilization and regulation of its phosphatase activity[22].

In addition to its ability to dephosphorylate protein, PTEN/MMAC1 can also dephosphorylate phosphatidylinositol (3,4,5)-triphosphate $(PI(3,4,5)P_3)$ at the D3 position of the inositol ring *in vitro*[23,24]. This has raised the question whether PTEN/MMAC1 exerts its action in part through regulation of the phosphoinositol pathway. $PI(3,4,5)P_3$ is a major lipid second messenger that is generated by the action of phosphoinositide 3-kinase (PI3K). $PI(3,4,5)P_3$ regulates a number of downstream effector pathways, including the oncoprotein Akt or protein kinase B (Akt/PKB) that is an important negative regulator of apoptosis and growth stimulation. Accordingly, absence of PTEN/MMAC1 and accumulation of $PI(3,4,5)P_3$ could lead to increased cellular proliferation and increased survival as discussed in more detail below.

The crystal structure of the PTEN/MMAC1 tumor suppressor has been established and allows a more thorough examination of its potential roles as a lipid and dual specificity phosphatase[21]. The phosphatase domain is very similar to other protein phosphatases, but the active site is enlarged, allowing for the accommodation of the $PI(3,4,5)P_3$ substrate. Mutations of Thr_{167} and Gln_{171} in the Tl loop within the active site diminished the $PI(3,4,5)P_3$ phosphatase activity by 60 and 75%, respectively. These amino acids form part of the binding pocket extension and the reduction in activity suggests that these residues are important of substrate binding. Mutations of the basic residues Lys_{125} and Lys_{128} resulted in large reductions in lipid phosphatase activity, confirming the model based on the crystal structure, indicating that these residues interact with the phosphates at $PI(3,4,5)P_3$ D1 and D5 residues, respectively.

The C-terminal 170 amino acids containing the C2 domain has a structure which is similar to those mediating Ca2+-dependent membrane recruitment of other signalling proteins, including PI3K, protein kinase C (PKC) and phopshoinositide-specific phospholipase C 1 (PLC 1)[21]. This structure consists of two antiparallel sheets with two short helices between the strands that forms a sandwich. This topology is similar to the C2 domains of PLC 1, PKC, and phospholipase A2. However, the PTEN/MMAC1 C2 domain lacks two of the three loops that comprise the Ca2+ binding sites in these proteins, suggesting that it may not bind membranes in a Ca2+-dependent manner. Nevertheless, the structure of the third loop (CBR3), which plays an important role in membrane binding has many features that are similar to Ca2+-dependent membrane binding proteins, suggesting that this region has a possible role in membrane association. Indeed, the PTEN/MMAC1 C2 domain was shown to have an affinity for phospholipid membranes *in vitro* that was independent of Ca2+[21]. Mutation of the C2 CBR3 region and subsequent expression in PTEN/MMAC1-deficient glioblastoma cells and comparison with wild-type PTEN/MMAC1-expressing cells indicated that cells expressing the mutants showed a higher proliferative index and lacked the comparable contact inhibition from the wild-type-expressing cells[21]. Since these mutants had comparable phosphatase activity as wild-type PTEN/MMAC1, the data indicate that the lipid binding function is important for the tumor suppressor activity.

To gain insight into the physiological actions of PTEN/MMAC1 studies of knock-out mice have been performed in several laboratories via homologous recombination that involved the removal of exons 3-5[25], 5[26] or 4 and 5[27]. All of these mutations remove the phosphatase catalytic domain, generating loss-of-function mutants of PTEN/MMAC1 that are similar to some of the mutations in CD patents. While some differences in phenotypes were observed in the 3 knock-out models that might be attributable to strain differences in the different mice, the overall results were generally similar. Homozygous deletion of the PTEN/MMAC1 gene resulted in embryonic lethality that occurred between 6.5 to 9.5 days, indicating an essential role for PTEN/MMAC1 in normal development. The hemizygous animals (PTEN/MMAC1[+/-]) were viable and exhibited a variety of hyperplastic-dysplastic changes in the prostate, skin and colon that are characteristic of CD, BZS and LDD. In addition, numerous other changes were observed, including, T cell lymphoma, lymphadenopathy or leukemia, radiation induced thymic lymphoma, teratocarcinoma, colon carcinomas, microscopic colonic hamartomas, gonadal stromal tumors, and hyperplastic thyroid or follicular/papillary thyroid neoplasia.

The developmental defects that occur in patients with CD, BZS and LDD is consistent with the important role for PTEN/MMAC1 that was observed in mouse embryogenesis. However, none of the mice had developmental abnormalities that directly mimicked those found in humans, including macrocephaly (CD), vascular malformations and speckled penis (BZS) or dysplastic gangliocytoma of the cerebellum (specific for LDD). These differences may indicate that PTEN/MMAC1 has differential roles in mouse and human development. Taken together these data suggest that PTEN/MMAC1 is not a canonical tumor suppressor gene, since all of the above changes appear to have occurred due to haploinsufficiency, although it cannot be ruled out that loss of the other allele occurred by mutation or gene silencing mechanisms. Importantly, the data provide direct support for the concept that PTEN/MMAC1 is a major tumor suppressor on chromosome 10q23 that is involved in the genesis and/or progression of a large number of cancers. These data do not necessarily rule out contributions of other tumor suppressor candidates such as *Mxi1* that is also located on chromosome 10q24, is frequently deleted in various cancers, and has been implicated in hyper-dysplastic features of the prostate in *Mxi1*[-/-] mice[28].

The fact that the different mouse knock-out models do display different phenotypes despite having a nearly identical knock-out strategy is of interest. For example, Podsypanina et al.[26] observed a striking phenotype of lymphadenopathy due to lymph node hyperplasia, which appears to be due to a deficit in apoptosis of the constituent cells of the lymph node. This was not observed in other models although these models did exhibit overt T cell lymphomas and/or T cell-derived leukemia[25,27]. Also, although Podsypanina et al.[26] observed intestinal tumors, these lacked the characteristic abnormalities of muscle or neural cell organization which are found in the human intestinal hamartomas with PTEN/MMAC1 mutations. By contrast, direct evidence for hamartomas was observed in the study of Suzuki et al.[25]. Indeed, the central role of a single gene such as PTEN/MMAC1 in mediating the different phenotypes in CD, BZS and LDD has been questioned. One possible explanation of these differences is that they may arise from differences in PTEN/MMAC1 gene dosage effects. Thus expression from the remaining wild-type allele could be controlled by other genetic factors, which could differ in the different mouse strains as well as the human backgrounds that lead to development of CD, BZS and LDD. Clearly, much effort will be required to sort out these more subtle developmental pathways and the potential role of gene dosage effects in mediating these events.

Mutations of the PTEN/MMAC1 Gene

Germline mutations of the PTEN/MMAC1 gene have been reported in several studies of CD, BZS, and LDD familes[29]. However, the finding of germline mutations in the PTEN/MMAC1 gene in juvenile polyposis coli, a disease that is also characterized by the development of hamartomas is controversial[30,31]. Of the mutations reported in CD and BZS, 26% represent frameshift mutations with the remainder representing point mutations comprising nonsense mutations (37%), missense mutation (25%) and bases substitutions that generate splice variants (13%). The majority (75%) of the germline mutations generate truncated proteins. Of the missense mutations 54% are clustered in the phosphatase core motif between residues 122 and 132 that resides in exon 5. A high proportion (54%) of the nonsense mutations reside in three positions: 130, 157, both in exon 5 and 233 in exon 7 of the PTEN/MMAC1 gene. Low frequency or absence of mutations in PTEN/MMAC1 gene has been reported in some CD and BZS patients[32-34], suggesting that the syndromes have a heterogeneous basis, but the evidence lies heavily in favor of the conclusion that the PTEN/MMAC1 gene is the susceptibility gene in CD and BZS.

Hemizygous deletion of the PTEN/MMAC1 gene occur very frequently in a variety of human tumors. Deletion rates can reach frequencies of 60-80 % in prostate cancer, advanced glial tumors and endometrial carcinoma. In addition, somatic mutations of the gene are also observed at very high rates in endometrial carcinomas (45%)[35-37], brain (24%)[38-40] and ovary (26%)[41,42]. Somatic mutations occur commonly at rates of 5-15% in a variety of other cancers, including, prostate, breast, head and neck, kidney, lung, melanoma, gastrointestinal tract and lymph[29]. With the high rates of deletion and mutation the PTEN/MMAC1 gene appears to be a classical tumor suppressor gene. However, given the marked gene dosage effect that is observed with the PTEN/MMAC1 gene in development[25-27], it is possible that gene dosage effects could also contribute to cancer development and/or progression.

PTEN/MMAC1 mutations have only been demonstrated in a minority of sporadic thyroid tumors, though these were detected more commonly in benign than malignant tumors (26% versus 6%), while loss of heterozygosity (LOH) in the PTEN/MMAC1 locus was also seen in 26% of the adenomas, but none of 10 follicular carcinomas. Our own data show similar results, with heterozygous PTEN/MMAC1 mutations detected in 29% of Hürthle cell follicular carcinomas, but no LOH in these same tumors, suggesting either that the

PTEN/MMAC1 gene is not involved in the development or progression of sporadic FTC, or that alternative means of gene silencing reduce its expression in these tumors. We[43] and others[44-46], have demonstrated frequent allelic imbalance in several chromosomal regions in FTC, most commonly involving 2p, 3p, 10q, 11q , and 17p,. At 10q, LOH centers on the 10q21-26 region[43,44]. PTEN/MMAC1 is therefore a strong candidate for the suspected 10q FTC tumor suppressor gene. However, when Dahia et al.[15] studied a group of 17 FTC, 39 PTC, 9 anaplastic thyroid carcinomas, and 30 follicular adenomas, they found a low frequency of LOH at the PTEN/MMAC1 locus, and could identify only a single PTEN/MMAC1 mutation in one PTC, despite the fact that PTC does not commonly exhibit LOH on 10q.

Since 10q LOH seems to be confined largely to follicular thyroid neoplasms, we analyzed tumor tissue from 14 patients with advanced FTC and 6 patients with benign follicular adenoma for PTEN/MMAC1 mutations and intragenic LOH. Ten FTC were of oxyphilic type, an aggressive variant[47], 11 were aneuploid and 4 were of pTNM stage III or IV. After a median of 6.4 years of follow up, 5 patients with FTC (36%) had died of thyroid cancer, resulting in a median survival time of 11.1 years. None of the tumors exhibited LOH at any of the three examined loci. One of the FTCs exhibited heterodimer formation of exon 8 on agarose gel electrophoresis, which subsequently was confirmed by sequencing to be due to a heterozygote 25 bp deletion. Dideoxy fingerprinting revealed possible mutations in 8 of the 180 amplified exons, affecting 7 FTC, but none of the FA. Somatic mutations were confirmed by DNA sequencing in 3 of these 7 FTC, for an overall PTEN/MMAC1 mutation rate of 21%. The mutations included nucleotide insertions, nucleotide substitutions, and microdeletions. In one case mutation resulted in a change in the exon 4 splice acceptor sequence, while the remaining mutations were predicted to result in prematurely terminated protein products. In all cases the other allele appeared to be the normal wild-type sequence. Thus our PTEN/MMAC1 mutation rate was higher than that reported previously in thyroid tumors by Dahia et al.[15], and more in line with published findings in other primary tumors[37,48-51], where the average PTEN/MMAC1 mutation rate is 15% (range 0%-62%). This result is consistent with our hypothesis that PTEN/MMAC1 mutations are seen more commonly in advanced FTC, and supports a role for this gene in disease progression.

PTEN/MMAC1 Mechanism of Action

The discrepancy between the relatively benign behavior of the neoplasms seen in Cowden Disease (germ-line mutations) and thyroid neoplasms (sporadic mutations), and the importance of PTEN/MMAC1 in the progression of advanced malignancies of other tissues, raises questions about its mechanism of action. While our understanding of the genetic basis of malignant disease is progressing rapidly, there remain fundamental questions to be addressed concerning the mechanism(s) by which these changes result in altered cell growth, proliferation and dissemination.

Phosphoinositide/Akt/PKB Pathway. The phosphoinositide pathway is very likely to represent the major pathway for regulation of PTEN/MMAC1 tumor suppressor function. Myers et al.[17] demonstrated that the missense mutation G129E that occurs in two CD kindreds, specifically ablates the ability of PTEN/MAC1 to recognize inositol phospholipids as a substrate. This suggests that loss of the lipid phosphatase, not the protein tyrosine phosphatase activity, is responsible for the genesis of CD. These authors went on to show that expression of wild-type or substrate-trapping forms of PTEN/MMAC1 in HEK293 cells altered the levels of the phospholipid products of PI3K. In addition, Myers et al.[17] identified Akt/PKB as a potential downstream effector of phospholipid products, since restoration of PTEN/MMAC1 expression in PTEN/MMAC1-deficient tumor cell lines inhibit Akt/PKB and affected cell survival.

$PI(3,4,5)P_3$ is the major product of PI3K that was initially discovered as a kinase activity that co-purified with the oncoproteins $pp60^{v\text{-}src}$ and polyoma middle T antigen[52]. Subsequently, it was discovered that the transforming ability of several oncoproteins was correlated with their ability to associate with PI3K. PI3K specifically phosphorylates the 3 position of the inositol ring and is also responsible for the generation of $PI(3,4)P_2$. Both $PI(3,4)P_2$ and $PI(3,4,5)P_3$ are found to increase dramatically upon oncoprotein transformation or growth factor stimulation, including platelet-derived growth factor, nerve growth factor and insulin-like growth factor 1. It is now known that $PI(3,4)P_2$ and $PI(3,4,5)P_3$ act as second messengers by the ability of certain proteins to bind to these lipids and become activated. Binding to these substrates occurs at the pleckstrin homology (PH) domains that recognize the phosphoinositide head group[53]. Some examples of PH-containing protein kinases are Bruton's tyrosine kinase (BTK), glutamine repeat protein -1 (GRP-1), Akt/PKB and 3-phosphoinositide-dependent protein kinase-1 (PDK1). Accordingly, the ability of PTEN/MMAC1 to dephosphorylate $PI(3,4)P_2$ and

$PI(3,4,5)P_3$ places it a central point in the control of the second messengers for a variety of tyrosine kinase-dependent pathways.

Akt/PKB was initially described as a viral transformning oncoprotein (v-akt) and was subsequently isolated and cloned as a PKC homologue, designated PKB[54]. It was recognized to be regulated by the PI3K pathway in studies of PDGF activation of Akt/PKB in fibroblasts[54]. Akt/PKB is localized to the membrane through interaction with $PI(3,4)P_2$ and $PI(3,4,5)P_3$ via its PH domain[55]. In addition, PDK1, a serine-threonine kinase has been shown to colocalize with Akt/PKB and is involved in its activation through its ability to phosphorylate the activation loop of the exposed catalytic domain[56,57]. Akt has received a great deal of attention through its control of apoptotic pathways and role in cell survival. Activation of Akt is associated with increased cell survival and is therefore thought to provide a mechanism for cancer progression. As depicted in Figure 2, Akt is thought to exert its antiapoptotic action by phosphorylating key members of the apoptotic pathway, including members of the forkhead family of transcription factors (FKHR)[58-60], the proapoptotic proteins BAD[61-63] and caspase-9[64]. The FKHR family members are homologs of a *Caenorhabditis elegans* factor designated DAF-16, itself a homolog of PTEN/MMAC1, which are downstream targets of two Akt homologs in an insulin-related signaling pathway[65-67]. Expression of active Akt can suppress human FKHR-mediated transcriptional activation by phosphorylation of three phosphoacceptor sites[68]. Mutation of these sites enhances the transcriptional activity of FKHR and renders it resistant to inhibition by Akt. Expression of the mutant FKHR in 293T results in apoptosis, suggesting that the FKHR family may be target for Akt/PKB that influences cell survival pathways. Akt is also involved in blocking cytochrome c release from mitochondria, an important event in the initiation of apoptosis as well as Fas-mediated apoptosis.

Akt/PKB may influence cellular proliferation through its ability to regulate the levels of $p27^{kip1}$, a potent cyclin/cyclin-dependent kinase (cdk) inhibitor[69] and its ability to phosphorylate and inactivate glycogen synthase kinase-3 (GSK-3)[70-72]. GSK-3 inactivation by Ak/tPKB phosphorylation leads to the stabilization of cylin D1 that can lead to cell cycle progression. Restoration of wild-type PTEN/MMAC1 in glioblastoma, breast and renal carcinoma cells that lack PTEN results in G1 arrest[73], which is accompanied by a posttranscriptional upregulation of $p27^{kip1}$. These effects can be mimicked by the PI3K inhibitors wortmannin and LY294002. That the effects of PTEN/MMAC1 expression in these cells are regulated by Akt/PKB is supported by the finding that coexpression of PTEN/MMAC1 with activated PI3K or Akt/PKB abrogated the growth inhibitory effects.

Focal Adhesion/ p125^FAK/Shc Pathway. Interest in the possibility that PTEN/MMAC1 might be involved in focal adhesion signalling was raised by the N-terminal domain homology that PTEN/MMAC1 shares with tensin[9,10,18]. Tensin is an SH2-containing protein that is involved in focal adhesion signal transduction pathways[74]. Focal adhesions represent structures that are formed when cells make contact with the extracellular matrix and formation of these structures is mediated by members of the integrin family. While such adhesions were originally thought to provide structural support for the cell s actin cytoskeleton, more recent studies have demonstrated that the focal adhesions are centers of intracellular signal transduction. In addition to tensin, other focal adhesion proteins involved in these processes include $p125^{FAK}$, Src family kinase, -actinin, talin, paxillin and $p130^{Cas}$. Other factors include growth factor receptors, mitogen-activated protein (MAP) kinase, Ras, NF- B , PI3K, PKC, IRS-1, caveolin-1 and c-Jun amino terminal kinase (JNK). The interactions of these focal adhesion proteins may be altered during cellular transformation. Accordingly, current interest focuses on the focal adhesion pathways and their influence on neoplastic transformation as well as cell spreading, migration, and invasion.

The integrins form an extensive family that is composed of pairs of at least 16 and subunits[75]. Different combinations of the subunits allow the formation of about 20 different heterodimeric receptors which span the plasmalemma. The extracellular portions of the integrin receptors interact with specific sites of the extracellular matrix proteins and these interactions are accompanied by receptor clustering that are essential for mediating intracellular responses. One of the proximal events in integrin-mediated signalling is the tyrosine phosphorylation of $p125^{FAK}$, which binds to the cytoplasmic domain of the integrin β_1 subunit[76]. Integrins can also interaction cooperatively with growth factors, cytokines and other serine/threonine kinases to provide multifunctional signalling opportunities[77-79]. Integrins can have complex effects on cell function, including both positive and negative contributions to the transformed phenotype. The integrin $\alpha_V\beta_3$ has been well documented to exhibit a positive influence on tumor proliferation and progression and is associated with increased malignancy in melanomas[80,81], while high level expression of integrin $\alpha_5\beta_1$ is associated decreased transformation and tumor formation[82,83]. Integrin-mediated activation of cell growth may be linked to the regulation of cycling and cyclin-dependent kinases and is thought to depend upon $p125^{FAK}$, since over-expression of FAK accelerates the G1 to S-phase transion and dominant-negative FAK mutants inhibit cell cycle progression at G1 as does microinjection of anit-FAK antibodies[84,85]. In some instances, proliferative responses of integrins may be mediated by Shc, the Src homology 2-containing protein adapters that link tyrosine kinases to Ras signaling through the Grb-2-Sos complex[86,87]. Figure 3 depicts a simplified version of this signalling cascade.

These integrin signalling pathways are also linked to apoptotic pathways, since many mammalian cells are dependent on extracellular matrix for survival and undergo anoikis (cell detachment-induced apoptosis) in the absence of a suitable matrix substrate[88]. Many tumor cells lose their dependence on anchorage to the extracellular matrix. Shc is thought to play a role in cell survival, since integrins that do not interact with Shc produce adhesion which is accompanied by cell cycle arrest and apoptosis that may be induced by JNK activation, which occurs early after extracellular matrix detachment[89,90]. However, FAK has also been implicated in promoting cell survival signals from the extracellular matrix. Expression of dominant-negative FAK mutants in cultured fibroblasts results in cycle arrest and apoptosis and similar results obtain upon microinjection of anit-FAK antibodies[85]. The p85 subunit of PI3K is associated with residue 397 of FAK upon attachment of cells to the extracellular matrix. This leads to rapid elevation of $PI(3,4)P_2$ and $PI(3,4,5)P_3$ with resultant activation of Akt/PKB and increased cell survival[91,92]. Also, constitutively active forms of FAK and/or PI3K protects cells from apoptosis in the absence of a suitable extracellular matrix[88,91]. PTEN/MMAC1 can therefore be seen as potentially having a dual role in the regulation of adhesion-mediated signalling. First, PTEN/MMAC1 may directly regulate FAK activity its ability to dephosphorylate FAK tyrosine phosphate[19,93]. Finally, through its ability to dephosphorylate $PI(3,4)P_2$ and $PI(3,4,5)P_3$ PTEN/MMAC1 may uncouple the FAK-mediated activation of the Akt/PKB pathway which is linked by PI3K.

Acknowledgements

This work was supported in part by National Institutes of Health grant DK80117 and by the Mayo Foundation Endocrine Neoplasia Program

Bibliography

1. Lloyd KM, Dennis M (1963) Cowden's disease A possible new symptom complex with multiple system involvement. Ann Intern Med 58:136-142.
2. Weary PE, Gorlin RJ, Gentry WC,Jr., Comer JE, Greer KE (1972) Multiple hamartoma syndrome (Cowden's disease). Arch Dermatol 106:682-690.
3. Hanssen AM, Fryns JP (1995) Cowden syndrome. J Med Genet 32:117-119.
4. Mallory SB (1995) Cowden syndrome (multiple hamartoma syndrome). Dermatol Clinics 13:27-31.
5. Harach HR, Soubeyran I, Brown A, Bonneau D, Longy M (1999) Thyroid pathologic findings in patients with Cowden disease. Ann Diagnos Pathol 3:331-340.
6. Brownstein MH, Mehregan AH, Bikowski JB, Lupulescu A, Patterson JC (1979) The dermatopathology of Cowden's syndrome. Br J Dermatol 100:667-673.
7. Alsanea O, Clark OH (2001) Familial thyroid cancer. Curr Opinion Oncol 13:44-51.
8. Nelen MR, Padberg GW, Peeters EA, et al (1996) Localization of the gene for Cowden disease to chromosome 10q22-23. Nature Genetics 13:114-116.
9. Li J, Yen C, Liaw D, et al (1997) PTEN, a putative protein tyrosine phosphatase gene mutated in human brain, breast, and prostate cancer. Science 275:1943-1947.
10. Steck PA, Pershouse MA, Jasser SA, et al (1997) Identification of a candidate tumour suppressor gene, MMAC1, at chromosome 10q23.3 that is mutated in multiple advanced cancers. Nature Genetics 15:356-362.
11. Liaw D, Marsh DJ, Li J, et al (1997) Germline mutations of the PTEN gene in Cowden disease, an inherited breast and thyroid cancer syndrome. Nature Genetics 16:64-67.

12. Nelen MR, van Staveren WC, Peeters EA, et al (1997) Germline mutations in the PTEN/MMAC1 gene in patients with Cowden disease. Hum Mol Genet 6:1383-1387.

13. Bonneau D, Longy M (2001) Mutations of the human PTEN gene. Human Mutation 16:109-122.

14. Chi SG, Kim HJ, Park BJ, et al (1998) Mutational abrogation of the PTEN/MMAC1 gene in gastrointestinal polyps in patients with Cowden disease. Gastroenterology 115:1084-1089.

15. Dahia PL, Marsh DJ, Zheng Z, et al (1997) Somatic deletions and mutations in the Cowden disease gene, PTEN, in sporadic thyroid tumors. Cancer Res 57:4710-4713.

16. Gimm O, Perren A, Weng LP, et al (2001) Differential nuclear and cytoplasmic expression of PTEN in normal thyroid tissue, and benign and malignant epithelial thyroid tumors. Am J Pathol 156:1693-1700.

17. Myers MP, Pass I, Batty IH, et al (1998) The lipid phosphatase activity of PTEN is critical for its tumor supressor function. Proc Natl Acad Sci USA 95:13513-13518.

18. Li DM, Sun H (1998) PTEN/MMAC1/TEP1 suppresses the tumorigenicity and induces G1 cell cycle arrest in human glioblastoma cells. Proc Natl Acad Sci USA 95:15406-15411.

19. Tamura M, Gu J, Matsumoto K, Aota S, Parsons R, Yamada KM (1998) Inhibition of cell migration, spreading, and focal adhesions by tumor suppressor PTEN. Science 280:1614-1617.

20. Ungewickell E, Ungewickell H, Holstein SE (1997) Functional interaction of the auxilin J domain with the nucleotide- and substrate-binding modules of Hsc70. J Biol Chem 272:19594-19600.

21. Lee JO, Yang H, Georgescu MM, et al (1999) Crystal structure of the PTEN tumor suppressor: implications for its phosphoinositide phosphatase activity and membrane association. Cell 99:323-334.

22. Vazquez F, Ramaswamy S, Nakamura N, Sellers WR (2001) Phosphorylation of the PTEN tail regulates protein stability and function. Molecular & Cellular Biology 20:5010-5018.

23. Maehama T, Dixon JE (1999) PTEN: a tumour suppressor that functions as a phospholipid phosphatase. Trends Cell Biol 9:125-128.

24. Maehama T, Dixon JE (1998) The tumor suppressor, PTEN/MMAC1, dephosphorylates the lipid second messenger, phosphatidylinositol 3,4,5-trisphosphate. J Biol Chem 273:13375-13378.

25. Suzuki A, de la Pompa JL, Stambolic V, et al (1998) High cancer susceptibility and embryonic lethality associated with mutation of the PTEN tumor suppressor gene in mice. Current Biology 8:1169-1178.

26. Podsypanina K, Ellenson LH, Nemes A, et al (1999) Mutation of Pten/Mmac1 in mice causes neoplasia in multiple organ systems. Proc Natl Acad Sci USA 96:1563-1568.

27. Di Cristofano A, Pesce B, Cordon-Cardo C, Pandolfi PP (1998) Pten is essential for embryonic development and tumour suppression. Nature Genetics 19:348-355.

28. Eagle LR, Yin X, Brothman AR, Williams BJ, Atkin NB, Prochownik EV (1995) Mutation of the MXI1 gene in prostate cancer. Nature Genetics 9:249-255.

29. Ali IU, Schriml LM, Dean M (1999) Mutational spectra of PTEN/MMAC1 gene: a tumor suppressor with lipid phosphatase activity. J Natl Cancer Inst 91:1922-1932.

30. Marsh DJ, Roth S, Lunetta KL, et al (1997) Exclusion of PTEN and 10q22-24 as the susceptibility locus for juvenile polyposis syndrome. Cancer Res 57:5017-5021.

31. Olschwang S, Serova-Sinilnikova OM, Lenoir GM, Thomas G (1998) PTEN germ-line mutations in juvenile polyposis coli. Nature Genetics 18:12-14.

32. Tsou HC, Teng DH, Ping XL, et al (1997) The role of MMAC1 mutations in early-onset breast cancer: causative in association with Cowden syndrome and excluded in BRCA1-negative cases. Am J Human Genet 1997; 61:1036-1043.

33. Nelen MR, Kremer H, Konings IB, et al (1999) Novel PTEN mutations in patients with Cowden disease: absence of clear genotype-phenotype correlations. Eur J Human Genet 7:267-273.

34. Carethers JM, Furnari FB, Zigman AF, et al (1998) Absence of PTEN/MMAC1 germ-line mutations in sporadic Bannayan-Riley-Ruvalcaba syndrome. Cancer Res 58:2724-2726.

35. Tashiro H, Isacson C, Levine R, Kurman RJ, Cho KR, Hedrick L(1997) p53 gene mutations are common in uterine serous carcinoma and occur early in their pathogenesis. Am J Pathol 150:177-185.

36. Tashiro H, Blazes MS, Wu R, et al (1997) Mutations in PTEN are frequent in endometrial carcinoma but rare in other common gynecological malignancies. Cancer Res 57:3935-3940.

37. Risinger JI, Hayes AK, Berchuck A, Barrett JC (1997) PTEN/MMAC1 mutations in endometrial cancers. Cancer Res 57:4736-4738.

38. Liu W, James CD, Frederick L, Alderete BE, Jenkins RB (1997) PTEN/MMAC1 mutations and EGFR amplification in glioblastomas. Cancer Res 57:5254-5257.

39. Zhou XP, Li YJ, Hoang-Xuan K, et al (1999) Mutational analysis of the PTEN gene in gliomas: molecular and pathological correlations. Int J Cancer 84:150-154.

40. Teng DH, Hu R, Lin H, et al (1997) MMAC1/PTEN mutations in primary tumor specimens and tumor cell lines. Cancer Res 57:5221-5225.

41. Yokomizo A, Tindall DJ, Hartmann L, Jenkins RB, Smith DI, Liu W (1998) Mutation analysis of the putative tumor suppressor PTEN/MMAC1 in human ovarian cancer. Int J Oncology 13:101-105.

42. Obata K, Morland SJ, Watson RH, Hitchcock A, Chenevix-Trench G, Campbell IG (1998) Frequent PTEN/MMAC mutations in endometrioid but not serous or mucinous epithelial ovarian tumors. Cancer Res 58:2095-2097.

43. Grebe SK, McIver B, Hay ID, et al (1997) Frequent loss of heterozygosity on chromosomes 3p and 17p without VHL or p53 mutations suggests involvement of unidentified tumor suppressor genes in follicular thyroid carcinoma. J Clin Endocrinol Metab 82:3684-3691.

44. Zedenius J, Wallin G, Svensson A, et al (1995) Allelotyping of follicular thyroid tumors. Human Genetics 96:27-32.

45. Tung WS, Shevlin DW, Kaleem Z, Tribune DJ, Wells SA,Jr, GoodfellowPJ (1997) Allelotype of follicular thyroid carcinomas reveals genetic instability consistent with frequent nondisjunctional chromosomal loss. Genes,Chromosomes & Cancer 19:43-51.

46. Ward LS, Brenta G, Medvedovic M, Fagin JA (1998) Studies of allelic loss in thyroid tumors reveal major differences in chromosomal instability between papillary and follicular carcinomas. J Clin Endocrinol Metab 83:525-530.

47. Grebe SK, Hay ID (1997) Follicular cell-derived thyroid carcinomas. Cancer Treat Res 89:91-140.

48. Cairns P, Okami K, Halachmi S, et al (1997) Frequent inactivation of PTEN/MMAC1 in primary prostate cancer. Cancer Res 57:4997-5000.

49. Guldberg P, thor Straten P, Birck A, Ahrenkiel V, Kirkin AF, ZeuthenJ (1997) Disruption of the MMAC1/PTEN gene by deletion or mutation is a frequent event in malignant melanoma. Cancer Res 57:3660-3663.

50. Wang SI, Puc J, Li J, et al (1997) Somatic mutations of PTEN in glioblastoma multiforme. Cancer Res 57:4183-4186.

51. Okami K, Wu L, Riggins G, et al (1998) Analysis of PTEN/MMAC1 alterations in aerodigestive tract tumors. Cancer Res 58:509-511.

52. Thompson DM, Cochet C, Chambaz EM, Gill GN (1985) Separation and characterization of a phosphatidylinositol kinase activity that co-purifies with the epidermal growth factor receptor. J Biol Chem 260:8824-8830.

53. Ferguson KM, Kavran JM, Sankaran VG, et al (2001) Structural basis for discrimination of 3-phosphoinositides by pleckstrin homology domains. Mol Cell 6:373-384.

54. Burgering BM, Coffer PJ (1995) Protein kinase B (c-Akt) in phos-phatidylinositol-3-OH kinase signal transduction. Nature 376:599-602.

55. Frech M, Andjelkovic M, Ingley E, Reddy KK, Falck JR, Hemmings BA. High affinity binding of inositol phosphates and phosphoinositi-des to the pleckstrin homology domain of RAC/protein kinase B and their influence on kinase activity. J Biol Chem 1997; 272:8474-8481.

56. Alessi DR, James SR, Downes CP, Holmes AB, Gaffney PR, Reese CB (1997) Characterization of a 3-phosphoinositide-dependent protein kinase which phosphorylates and activates protein kinase Balpha. Current Biology 7:261-269.

57. Stephens L, Anderson K, Stokoe D, et al (1998) Protein kinase B kinases that mediate phosphatidylinositol 3,4,5-trisphosphate-dependent activation of protein kinase B. Science 279:710-714.

58. Uddin S, Kottegoda S, Stigger D, Platanias LC, Wickrema A (2001) Activation of the Akt/FKHRL1 pathway mediates the antiapoptotic effects of erythropoietin in primary human erythroid progenitors. Biochem Biophys Res Comm 275:16-19.

59. Kashii Y, Uchida M, Kirito K, et al (2001) A member of Forkhead family transcription factor, FKHRL1, is one of the downstream molecules of phosphatidylinositol 3-kinase-Akt activation pathway in erythropoietin signal transduction. Blood 96:941-949.

60. del Peso L, Gonzalez VM, Hernandez R, Barr FG, Nunez G (1999) Regulation of the forkhead transcription factor FKHR, but not the PAX3-FKHR fusion protein, by the serine/threonine kinase Akt. Oncogene 18:7328-7333.

61. Graff JR, Konicek BW, McNulty AM, et al (2001) Increased AKT activity contributes to prostate cancer progression by dramatically accelerating prostate tumor growth and diminishing p27Kip1 expression. J Biol Chem 275:24500-24505.

62. Tang Y, Zhou H, Chen A, Pittman RN, Field J (2001) The Akt proto-oncogene links Ras to Pak and cell survival signals. J Biol Chem 275:9106-9109.

63. Hunter MG, Avalos BR (2001) Granulocyte colony-stimulating factor receptor mutations in severe congenital neutropenia transforming to acute myelogenous leukemia confer resistance to apoptosis and enhance cell survival. Blood 95:2132-2137.

64. Cardone MH, Roy N, Stennicke HR, et al (1998) Regulation of cell death protease caspase-9 by phosphorylation. Science 282:1318-1321.

65. Ayala JE, Streeper RS, Desgrosellier JS, et al (1999) Conservation of an insulin response unit between mouse and human glucose-6-phosphatase catalytic subunit gene promoters: transcription factor FKHR binds the insulin response sequence. Diabetes 48:1885-1889.

66. Guo S, Rena G, Cichy S, He X, Cohen P, Unterman T (1999) Phosphorylation of serine 256 by protein kinase B disrupts transactivation by FKHR and mediates effects of insulin on insulin-like growth factor-binding protein-1 promoter activity through a conserved insulin response sequence. J Biol Chem 274:17184-17192.

67. Rytomaa M, Lehmann K, Downward J (2001) Matrix detachment induces caspase-dependent cytochrome c release from mitochondria: inhibition by PKB/Akt but not Raf signalling. Oncogene 19:4461-4468.

68. Tang ED, Nunez G, Barr FG, Guan KL (1999) Negative regulation of the forkhead transcription factor FKHR by Akt. J Biol Chem 274:16741-16746.

69. Collado M, Medema RH, Garcia-Cao I, et al (2001) Inhibition of the phosphoinositide 3-kinase pathway induces a senescence-like arrest mediated by p27Kip1. J Biol Chem 275:21960-21968.

70. Gold MR, Scheid MP, Santos L, et al (1999) The B cell antigen receptor activates the Akt (protein kinase B)/glycogen synthase kinase-3

signaling pathway via phosphatidylinositol 3-kinase. J Immunol 163:1894-1905.

71. Lavoie L, Band CJ, Kong M, Bergeron JJ, Posner BI (1999) Regulation of glycogen synthase in rat hepatocytes. Evidence for multiple signaling pathways. J Biol Chem 274:28279-28285.

72. Cross DA, Alessi DR, Cohen P, Andjelkovich M, Hemmings BA (1995) Inhibition of glycogen synthase kinase-3 by insulin mediated by protein kinase B. Nature 378:785-789.

73. Lu Y, Lin YZ, LaPushin R, et al (1999) The PTEN/MMAC1/TEP tumor suppressor gene decreases cell growth and induces apoptosis and anoikis in breast cancer cells. Oncogene 18:7034-7045.

74. Weisberg E, Sattler M, Ewaniuk DS, Salgia R (1997) Role of focal adhesion proteins in signal transduction and oncogenesis. Crit Rev Onogenesis 8:343-358.

75. Schwartz MA (1997) Integrins, oncogenes, and anchorage independence. J Cell Biol 139:575-578.

76. Lewis JM, Schwartz MA (1995) Mapping *in vivo* associations of cytoplasmic proteins with integrin beta 1 cytoplasmic domain mutants. Mol Biol Cell 6:151-160.

77. McNamee HP, Ingber DE, Schwartz MA (1993) Adhesion to fibronectin stimulates inositol lipid synthesis and enhances PDGF-induced inositol lipid breakdown. J Cell Biol 121:673-678.

78. Arora PD, Ma J, Min W, Cruz T, McCulloch CA (1995) Interleukin-1-induced calcium flux in human fibroblasts is mediated through focal adhesions. J Biol Chem 270:6042-6049.

79. Renshaw MW, Ren XD, Schwartz MA (1997) Growth factor activation of MAP kinase requires cell adhesion. EMBO J 16:5592-5599.

80. Felding-Habermann B, Mueller BM, Romerdahl CA, Cheresh DA (1992) Involvement of integrin alpha V gene expression in human melanoma tumorigenicity. J Clin Invest 89:2018-2022.

81. Albelda SM, Mette SA, Elder DE, Stewart R, Damjanovich L, Herlyn M (1990) Integrin distribution in malignant melanoma: association of the beta 3 subunit with tumor progression. Cancer Res 50:6757-6764.

82. Schreiner C, Fisher M, Hussein S, Juliano RL (1991) Increased tumorigenicity of fibronectin receptor deficient Chinese hamster ovary cell variants. Cancer Res 51:1738-1740.

83. Giancotti FG, Ruoslahti E (1990) Elevated levels of the alpha 5 beta 1 fibronectin receptor suppress the transformed phenotype of Chinese hamster ovary cells. Cell 60:849-859.

84. Gilmore AP, Romer LH (1996) Inhibition of focal adhesion kinase (FAK) signaling in focal adhesions decreases cell motility and proliferation. Mol Biol Cell 7:1209-1224.

85. Zhao JH, Reiske H, Guan JL (1998) Regulation of the cell cycle by focal adhesion kinase. J Cell Biol 143:1997-2008.

86. Vuori K, Ruoslahti E (1993) Activation of protein kinase C precedes alpha 5 beta 1 integrin-mediated cell spreading on fibronectin. J Biol Chem 268:21459-21462.

87. Wary KK, Mariotti A, Zurzolo C, Giancotti FG (1998) A requirement for caveolin-1 and associated kinase Fyn in integrin signaling and anchorage-dependent cell growth. Cell 94:625-634.

88. Frisch SM, Vuori K, Ruoslahti E, Chan-Hui PY (1996) Control of adhesion-dependent cell survival by focal adhesion kinase. J Cell Biol 134:793-799.

89. Frisch SM, Vuori K, Kelaita D, Sicks S (1996) A role for Jun-N-terminal kinase in anoikis; suppression by bcl-2 and crmA. J Cell Biol 135:1377-1382.

90. Wary KK, Mainiero F, Isakoff SJ, Marcantonio EE, Giancotti FG (1996) The adaptor protein Shc couples a class of integrins to the control of cell cycle progression. Cell 87:733-743.

91. Khwaja A, Rodriguez-Viciana P, Wennstrom S, Warne PH, Downward J (1997) Matrix adhesion and Ras transformation both activate a phosphoinositide 3-OH kinase and protein kinase B/Akt cellular survival pathway. EMBO J 16:2783-2793.

92. Chen HC, Guan JL (1994) Association of focal adhesion kinase with its potential substrate phosphatidylinositol 3-kinase. Proc Natl Acad Sci USA 91:10148-10152.

93. Tamura M, Gu J, Takino T, Yamada KM (1999) Tumor suppressor PTEN inhibition of cell invasion, migration, and growth: differential involvement of focal adhesion kinase and p130Cas. Cancer Res 59:442-449.

Tablel 1. International Cowden Consortium Diagnostic Criteria.

Diagnosis by Mucocutaneous Lesions (Any one of the following:)
Six or more papules, at least three of which are trichilemmomas.
Cutaneous facial papules plus oral papillomatosis.
Oral papillomatosis plus acral keratoses.
Six or more palmoplantar keratoses.

Pathognomonic Mucocutaneous Lesions
Multiple facial trichilemmomas (tumors of the follicular infundibulum, resembling flesh-colored veruccous warts).
Acral keratoses (hyperkarototic papules on the dorsal surfaces of the extremities and palmoplantar keratoses).
Papillomatous lesions.
Oral lesions of gingival and buccal mucosa and tongue.

Dignaosis by Non-mucocutaneous Criteria
Lhermitte-Duclos disease and thyroid or breast cancer.
Macrocephaly and thyroid or breast cancer.
One major criterion and three minor criteria.
Four minor criteria.

Major Criteria
Breast cancer.
Thyroid cancer.
Macrocephaly.
Lhermitte-Duclos disease.

Minor Criteria
Thyroid lesions.
Mental retardation (I.Q. < 75).
Gastrointestinal hamartomas.
bibrocystic disease of the breast.
Lipomas or fibromas.
Genitourinary tumors of malformations.

Table 2. Benign Features of Cowden Disease.

Thyroid	Breast	Genitourinary	GI Tract
Goiter Thyroiditis AITD Follicular Adenoma	Hypertrophy Fibrocystic Disease Gynecomastia	Irregular Menses Ovarian Cysts Testicular Hypoplasia	Diffuse Polyposis Diverticulae Hepati Hamar- tomas
Skeletal High-Arched Palate >Adenoid Faces= Pectus/ScoliosisBone Cysts	**CNS** Neuromas Neurofibromas Meningiomas	**Miscellaneous** Mental Retardation ASD Cataracts Pulmonary Hamar- tomas	

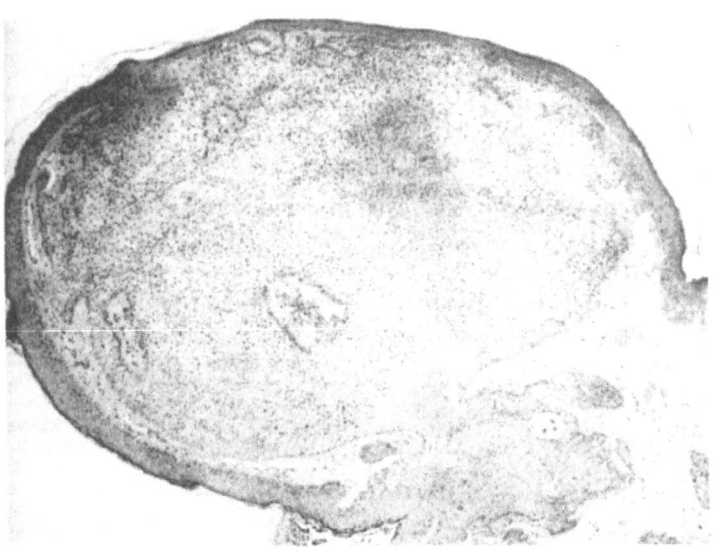

Figure 1. Characteristic dermatologic features of Cowden disease.

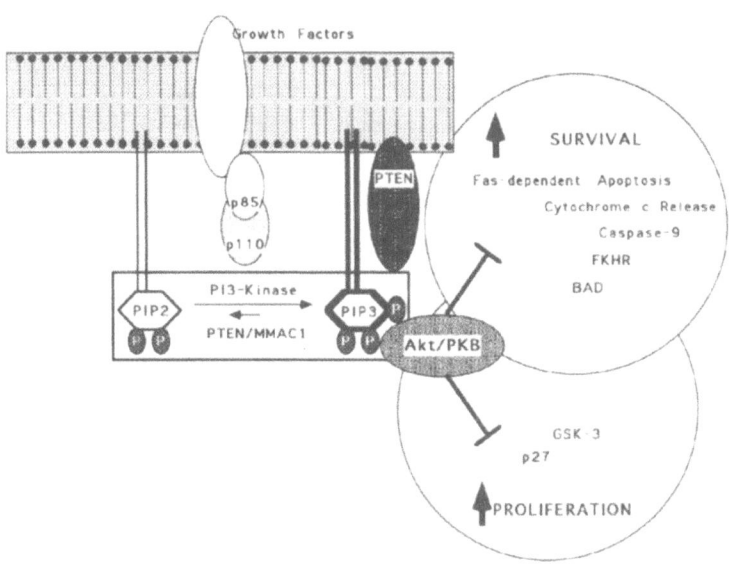

Figure 2. Schematic representation of mechanism of PTEN/MMAC1 action regulating growth factor-mediated pathways,through its action as a lipid phosphatase, controlling the lipid second messenger PI(3,4,5)P$_3$. Reduction of PTEN/MMAC1 activity results in the accumulation of PI(3,4,5)P$_3$, and consequent activation of Akt/PKB, which increases cell survival by inhibition of apoptosis and proliferation, through inactivation of GSK-3 and p27.

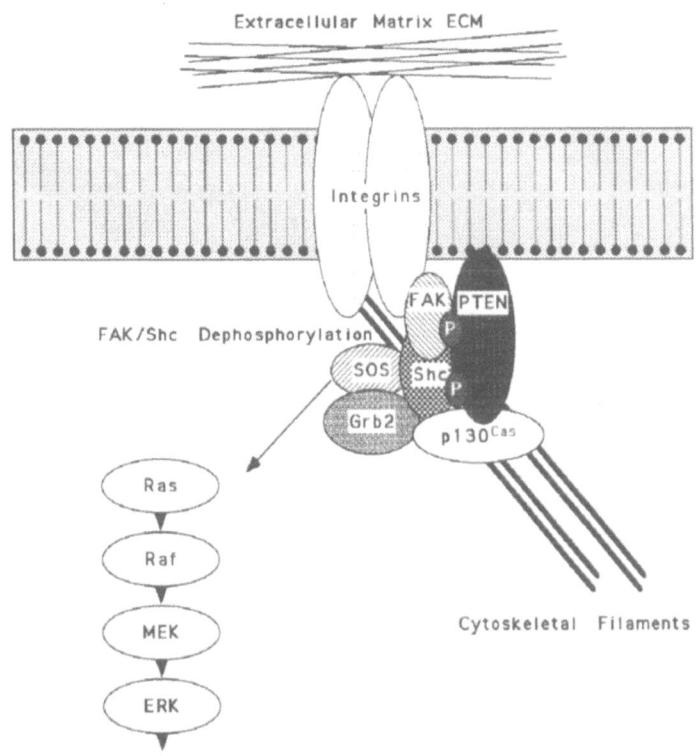

Figure 3. Schematic representation of mechanism of PTEN/MMAC1 action regulating adhesion-stimulated pathways, through its action as a protein phosphatase. Reduced activity of PTEN/MMAC1 permits sustained activation of the FAK/Shc-mediated activitiaon of the Ras/Raf/MEK cascade, promoting migration, invasion, and growth.

Molecular mechanisms of RET activation in human neoplasia

Massimo Santoro, Francesca Carlomagno, Rosa Marina Melillo,
Giancarlo Vecchio and Alfredo Fusco
Centro di Endocrinologia ed Oncologia Sperimentale del CNR c/o Dipartimento di Biologia e Patologia Cellulare e Molecolare, Facoltà di Medicina e Chirurgia, Università di Napoli "Federico II", via S. Pansini 5, 80131 Naples, Italy
Corresponding author: Massimo Santoro, Centro di Endocrinologia ed Oncologia Sperimentale del C.N.R., Università degli Studi di Napoli, via S. Pansini 5, 80131 Naples, Italy. Ph: 39.081.7463056; Fax: 39.081.7463037; Email: masantor@unina.it

Summary

Mutations that produce oncogenes with dominant gain of function may target receptor protein tyrosine kinases (PTK) in cancer and confer uncontrolled proliferation, impaired differentiation or unrestrained survival to the cancer cell. On the other hand, insufficient PTKs' signaling may be responsible for developmental diseases. Gain of function of the RET receptor PTK is associated to human cancer. At the germ line level, point mutations of RET are responsible for multiple endocrine neoplasia type 2 (MEN2A, MEN2B and FMTC). Mutations of extracellular cysteines are found in MEN2A patients and a Met918Thr mutation is responsible for MEN2B. At the somatic level, gene rearrangements juxtaposing the TK domain of RET to heterologous gene partners are found in papillary carcinomas of the thyroid. These rearrangements generate the chimeric RET/PTC oncogenes. Both MEN2-associated point mutations and PTC-associated gene rearrangements potentiate the intrinsic TK activity of RET and, ultimately, the RET downstream signaling events. A multidocking site of the C-tail of RET is essential for both mitogenic and survival RET signalling. Such a site is involved in the recruitment of several intracellular molecules, like the Shc, FRS2 and IRS1 docking proteins and Enigma. The different activating mutations may also alter qualitatively the RET signaling properties either by altering RET auto-phosphorylation (in the case of the MEN2B mutation) or the subcellular distribution of the active kinase or providing the active kinase with a scaffold for novel protein-protein interactions (as in the case of RET/PTC oncoproteins). This review describes the molecular mechanisms by which the different genetic alterations cause the conversion of RET into a dominant transforming oncogene.

Key words
protein tyrosine kinase, PTK, RET, multiple endocrine neoplasia, MEN, FMTC, PTC, medullary thyroid carcinoma

The RET receptor tyrosine kinase
RET is an evolutionary conserved gene; RET homologs have been found in human, mouse, rat, zebrafish and fruitfly. RET encodes a transmembrane receptor of the protein tyrosine kinase family (1). RET protein is composed by three domains: an extracellular domain which contains the signal peptide and cadherin-like and cysteine-rich regions; a transmembrane domain; an intracellular portion containing the tyrosine kinase domain (TK) splitted by the insertion of 27 aminoacids. RET is the receptor of growth factors belonging to the glial cell line derived neurotrophic factor (GDNF) family. This family comprises the GDNF, neurturin (NTN), persephin (PSP), and artemin, which all have trophic influences on a variety of neuronal populations (2). They interact with multimeric receptors composed by high-affinity glycosyl-phosphatidylinositol (GPI)-linked receptors and the RET kinase. Four GPI-linked co-receptors have been isolated and designated GFRα1, 2, 3 and 4. A preferential (in some cases exclusive) interaction of GDNF, NTN, artemin, and PSP with GFRα1, 2, 3 and 4, respectively, has been demonstrated. In turn, the ligand-coreceptor complex interacts with RET and induces dimerization and activation of the kinase and signal transduction. Ligand-dependent RET activation is able to promote neuronal cell survival and differentiation (2). Moreover, RET plays an essential role in kidney development. Accordingly, RET- and co-receptor- *null* mice show severe defects of the innervation of the hindgut and branching of the ureteric bud.

Oncogenic activation of RET in thyroid papillary carcinomas
Papillary thyroid carcinomas are frequently associated with specific alterations affecting the RET gene (3). These rearrangements lead to the fusion of the RET TK-encoding domain to the 5'-terminal regions of heterologous genes, generating chimeric oncogenes designated RET/PTC.

177

As illustrated in Fig. 1, several RET fusion partners have been isolated so far including the H4, RIα, and RFG genes in the case of RET/PTC1, 2, 3 (4-6). RET, H4 and RFG genes map on the long arm of chromosome 10 and their fusion is generated by chromosome inversions; RET/PTC2 is generated by a balanced translocation between chromosomes 10 and 17 (3).

Thyroid carcinomas are divided in differentiated (papillary and follicular) and undifferentiated (anaplastic) carcinoma (7). RET/PTC on-cogenes are found with a variable frequency (from 2.5 to 40%) in papillary carcinomas (8 and references herein). A high frequency of RET rearrangements is found in thyroid microcarcinomas, which are papillary tumors with low growing and invading tendency (9). RET/PTC rearrangements have never been found in tumors other than carcinomas of the thyroid gland (3). Ionizing radiations are able to induce RET/PTC rearrangements and thyroid cancer is the most common form of solid neoplasm associated with radiation exposure (10). Accordingly, a dramatic increase of the incidence of pediatric papillary carcinomas has been reported following the Chernobyl nuclear accident which released 50-200 million curies of radiation (11); RET/PTC rearrangements are highly prevalent in these carcinomas (12). RET/PTC are transforming oncogenes. They have been isolated by virtue of their ability of transforming NIH 3T3 fibroblasts, and they have been found to transform epithelial thyroid cells (13) and to induce papillary thyroid carcinomas in transgenic mice (14-15). These rearrangements activate the transforming potential of RET by multiple mechanisms. First, by substituting its transcriptional promoter with those of the fusion partners, they allow the expression of RET in the thyroid cells where it is normally transcriptionally silent. On the other side, the rearrangements generate constitutively active chimeric oncoproteins which are distributed in the cytosolic compartment of the cell. The activation of the RET kinase is mediated by the substitution of the extracellular portion with domains that are capable of mediating dimerization. In fact, RET fusion partners contain coiled-coil domains which are well-known protein-protein interaction motifs. At this time, it is still unknown which functional consequence, if any, may derive from the altered localization (from the plasmamembrane to the cytosol) of the RET kinase.

Oncogenic activation of RET in MEN2 syndromes

Germline point mutations of RET are responsible for the inheritance of the MEN2 familial tumoral syndromes and somatic mutations are found in a fraction of sporadic medullary thyroid carcinomas and pheochromocytomas. MEN2 are divided in three different clinical varieties: MEN2A, characterized by the presence of medullary thyroid carcinomas, pheocromocytomas and parathyroid hyperplasia; FMTC, in which medullary thyroid carcinoma is the only phenotype; MEN2B characterized by medullary thyroid carcinomas associated to phaeocromocytomas, enteric ganglioneuromas, and skeletal and ocular abnormalities (16). These clinical varieties are caused by different RET mutations falling into two main groups: those affecting the extracellular and those of the TK domain. MEN2A mutations cause the substitution of extracellular cysteines (609, 611, 618, 620, 630, 634) with several other residues (55-56). In particular, about 90% of MEN2A patients have a mutation of Cys634 and this mutation is highly predictive of the presence of pheochromocytoma and parathyroid hyperplasia. Two alternative mutations, one affecting residue 631 and another consisting in an insertion creating an additional cysteine, have been also described (16). FMTC mutations can be of the extracellular or the TK type. Extracellular FMTC mutations are similar to those causing MEN2A, but are more homogeneously distributed on cysteines 618, 620 and 634. Mutations of residues 768, 790, 791, 804, 844, or 891 of the RET TK domain have been also found in FMTC patients. Finally, MEN2B is caused by the highly specific Met918Thr (95%) or the Ala883Phe (3%) mutations. The Met918Thr substitution is the most frequently found mutation in sporadic medullary thyroid carcinomas (16).

All these point mutations have a "gain of function" effect. A constitutive dimerization is the molecular mechanism of the activation of RET molecules carrying mutations affecting extracellular cysteines (17). Although the three-dimensional structure of the RET extracellular domain is still unknown, it is likely that these cysteines form intramolecular disulfide bonds in the wild type receptor and that the mutation results in an unpaired cysteine which forms an activating inter-molecular bridge. A different intensity in the induction of the dimerization is a reasonable explanation for the phenotypes caused by mutations of the different cysteines. Indeed, RET mutants associated with FMTC have low dimerization and maturation efficiencies and this can explain why their kinase and oncogenic activities are lower than those of the classic MEN2A mutant.

MEN2B mutations cause a constitutive activation of the RET transforming potential. However, in addition to "quantitative" changes of the basal kinase activity, the most frequent MEN2B mutation (Met918Thr) is proposed to affect also the "quality" of RET-generated intracellular signals. The residue corresponding to RET methionine 918 is conserved in all receptor tyrosine kinases (RTK), while cytoplasmic protein tyrosine kinases (PTK) show a threonine in that position. This residue maps in the pocket of the kinase involved in substrate binding and, thus, it is predicted to alter the substrate selection (17). Thus, the molecular mechanism by which the Met918Thr mutation alters RET function is probably multiple. On one side, this mutation leads to a ligand-independent activation of the kinase without causing a constitutive dimerization of RET molecules. On the other side, the Met918Thr substitution modifies RET substrate specificity. This may result in an alteration of RET autophosphorylation sites as well as of the pattern of intracellular phosphorylated proteins. MEN2B kinase activity can be further enhanced by the ligand and this probably results in a stimulation which is stronger than that caused by the MEN2A mutation.

Concluding remarks

Somatic rearrangements, which, at the same time, substitute RET transcriptional promoter and cause an activation of the kinase, are selected in carcinomas deriving from follicular thyroid cells where RET is normally transcriptionally silent. The chronic activation of intracellular pathways downstream RET tyrosine kinase may specifically cause the papillary tumoral phenotype. On the other side, RET is normally expressed in tissues which are affected by the MEN2 syndromes. Alternative point mutations cause the different MEN2 phenotypes. The MEN2B disease is the most aggressive form of MEN2; its severe phenotype is probably explained by a combination of mechanisms including constitutive activation of the kinase, susceptibility to a further stimulation by the ligand and change of the signalling specificity. Several aspects of the molecular mechanisms of RET activation deserve further investigation. The role played by the RET fusion partners and by the delocalization of the kinase as well as the reason for the restriction of RET/PTC rearrangements to the thyroid gland still need to be clarified. A polyclonal hyperplasia of thyroid C-cells is the first result of the inheritance of a MEN2-type RET mutant and it is reasonable to think that further genetic events are required to induce the tumor phenotype. Whether RET has prevalently mitogenic, transforming or survival effects in its *in vivo* cell targets has yet to be ascertained; moreover, at this time, which are the intracellular signal transducers involved in these biological responses can only be hypothesized. It is already possible to identify MEN2 carriers through the analysis of germline DNA and on the basis of the genotype-phenotype correlation to program a differentiated treatment. Moreover, the identification of RET/PTC rearrangements may be of help in the differential diagnosis of follicular thyroid tumoral diseases. Finally, understanding the molecular basis of RET signalling will help attempting novel therapeutic strategies aimed to interfere with these pathways.

Acknowledgements

This study was supported by the Associazione Italiana per la Ricerca sul Cancro (AIRC), the Progetto Biotecnologie "5%" of the Consiglio Nazionale delle Ricerche (C.N.R.) and Progetto M.U.R.S.T. "Terapie antineoplastiche innovative". The paper was written while G. Vecchio was a Scholar-in-Residence at the Fogarty International Center for Advanced Study in the Health Sciences, National Institutes of Health, Bethesda.

References

1.   1. Takahashi M, Buma Y, Iwamoto T, Inaguma Y, Ikeda H, Hiai H (1988) Cloning and   expression of the ret protooncogene encoding a tyrosine kinase with two potential transmembrane domains. Oncogene 3: 571

2.   Robertson K, Mason I (1997) The GDNF-RET signalling partnership. Trends Genet. 13: 1

3.   Pierotti M.A, Bongarzone I, Borello M.G, Greco A, Pilotti S, Sozzi G (1996) Cytogenetics and molecular genetics of carcinomas arising from thyroid epithelial follicular cells. Genes Chrom. Cancer, 16: 1

4.   Grieco M, Santoro M, Berlingieri M.T, Melillo R.M, Donghi R, Bongarzone I, Pierotti M.A, Della Porta G, Fusco A, Vecchio G (1990) PTC is a novel rearranged form of the ret proto-oncogene and is frequently detected in vivo in human thyroid papillary carcinomas. Cell 60: 557

5.   Santoro M, Dathan N.A, Berlingieri M.T, Bongarzone I, Paulin C, Grieco M, Pierotti M.A, Vecchio G, Fusco A (1994) Molecular characterization of RET/PTC3: a novel rearranged version of the RET proto-oncogene in a human thyroid papillary carcinoma. Oncogene 9: 509

6.   Bongarzone I, Monzini N, Borrello M.G, Carcano C, Ferraresi G, Arighi E, Mondellini P, Della Porta G, Pierotti M.A (1993) Molecular characterization of a thyroid tumor-specific transforming sequence formed by the fusion of ret tyrosine kinase and the regulatory subunit RI alpha of cyclic AMP-dependent protein kinase A. Mol. Cell. Biol. 13: 358

7.   Hedinger C, Williams E.D, Sobin L.H (1989) The WHO histological classification of thyroid tumors: a commentary on the second edition. Cancer 63: 908

8.   Tallini G, Santoro M, Helie M, Carlomagno F, Salvatore G, Chiappetta G, Carcangiu M.L, Fusco A (1998) RET/PTC oncogene activation defines a subset of papillary thyroid carcinomas lacking evidence of progression to poorly differentiated or undifferentiated tumor phenotypes. Clin. Cancer Res 4: 287

9.   Viglietto G, Chiappetta G, Martinez-Tello FJ, Fukunaga FH, Tallini G, Rigopoulou D, Visconti R., Mastro A., Santoro M., Fusco A (1995) RET/PTC oncogene activation is an early event in thyroid carcinogenesis. Oncogene 11: 1207

10.   Williams E.D (1993) Radiation-induced thyroid cancer. Histopathology 23: 387

11.   Jacob P, Goulko G, Heidenreich W.F, Likhtarev I, Kairo I, Tronko N.D, Bogdanova T.I, Kenigsberg J, Buglova E, Drozdovitch V, Golovneva A, Demidchik E.P, Balonov M, Zvonova I, Beral V (1998) Thyroid cancer risk to children calculated. Nature 392: 31

12.   Fugazzola L, Pilotti S, Pinchera A, Vorontsova T.V, Mondellini P, Bongarzone I, Greco A, Astakhova L, Butti M.G, Demidchik E.P, Pacini F, Pierotti M.A (1995) Oncogenic rearrangements of the RET proto-oncogene in papillary thyroid carcinomas from children exposed to the Chernobyl nuclear accident. Cancer Res 55: 5617

13.   Santoro M, Melillo R.M, Grieco M, Berlingieri M.T, Vecchio G, Fusco A (1993) The TRK and RET tyrosine kinase oncogenes cooperate with ras in the neoplastic transformation of a rat thyroid epithelial cell line. Cell Growth Differ 4: 77

14.   Jhiang S.M, Sagartz J.E, Tong Q, Parker-Thornburg J, Capen C.C, Cho J.Y, Xing S, Ledent C (1996) Targeted expression of the ret/PTC1 oncogene induces papillary thyroid carcinomas. Endocrinology 137: 375

15.   Santoro M, Chiappetta G, Cerrato A, Salvatore D, Zhang L, Manzo G, Picone A, Portella G, Santelli G, Vecchio G, Fusco A (1996) Development of thyroid papillary carcinomas secondary to tissue-specific expression of the RET/PTC1 oncogene in transgenic mice. Oncogene 12: 1821

16.   Pasini B, Ceccherini I, Romeo G (1996) RET mutations in human disease. Trends Genet. 12: 138

17.   Santoro M, Carlomagno F, Romano A, Bottaro D.P, Dathan N.A, Grieco M, Fusco A, Vecchio G, Matoskova B, Kraus M.H, Di Fiore P.P (1995) Germ-line mutations of MEN2A and MEN2B activate RET as a dominant transforming gene by different molecular mechanisms. Science 267: 381

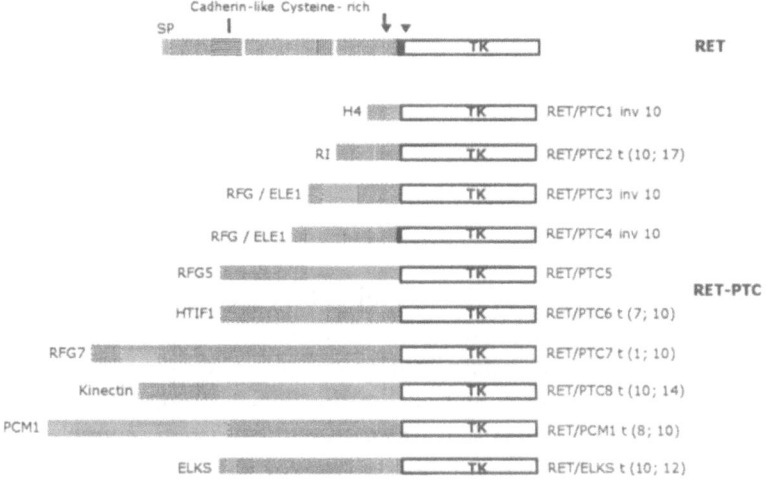

Figure 1

RET/PTC oncogenes, which are found in papillary thyroid carcinomas, are chimeric genes generated by the fusion of the RET tyrosine-kinase (TK) encoding domain to different heterologous genes

Lessons from Chernobyl; need for molecular epidemiology of childhood thyroid cancer

Shunichi Yamashita, Hiroyuki Namba, Noboru Takamura,
Kiyoto Ashizawa and Yoshisada Shibata
Atomic Bomb Disease Institute, Nagasaki University School of Medicine
1-12-4 Sakamoto Nagasaki 8528523,Japan
Tel; 81-95-849-7114 Fax; 81-95-849-7117
E-mail; shun@net.nagasaki-u.ac.jp

Abstract

The results of Chernobyl Sasakawa project have clearly demonstrated the comparable data of childhood thyroid diseases around Chernobyl under the same protocol and standardized procedures, indicating the highest number of thyroid nodules and cancers in Gomel region, Belarus. According to the results of the highest number of childhood thyroid cancer and the necessity of long-term follow-up for the high-risk group of childhood thyroid diseases, further studies have been conducted in these areas. The relationship has not been clarified between radiation-exposure and childhood thyroid diseases, especially low-dose radiation-exposure and thyroid cancer. Therefore the new Chernobyl Sasakawa project has been focused on the continuation of thyroid screening and epidemiological studies; cohort study and case-control study of childhood thyroid cancer in Belarus and in Russia, respectively, from May 1996 till April 2001. Furthermore, the comparative study have been in action in Gomel region for the children who were born before and after the Chernobyl accident, in order to clarify the vulnerable population and significant implication of short-live radioactive iodines on thyroid carcinogenesis fallen out just after the accident.

Based on the above results of Chernobyl Sasakawa project, ret/PTC gene rearrangement has been examined using the tissues obtained from

Chernobyl. Now many reports indicate the evidence of high incidence of ret/PTC gene rearrangement in childhood thyroid cancer tissues. To further clarify the in vitro molecular mechanism of radiation-induced thyroid specific carcinogenesis, p53 and other signal transduction involvement induced by radiation have been examined. The search for signature gene(s) and target molecules of radiation-associated thyroid carcningenesis is urgently needed. Our experimental results demonstrated that radiation-exposure could cause abnormal thyroid cell proliferation specifically through constitutive activation of intracellular target molecules and disturb the apoptosis-prone pathway, besides the direct genetic alteration.

Therefore, the late effect of radiation, even in the lower dose, on human thyroid glands should be monitored carefully for the radiation-sensitive vulnerable group at any radiocontaminated area for longer period.

Key words

Chernobyl, screening, thyroid cancer, oncogene, ret/PTC rearrangement, signal transduction

Introduction

Ionizing radiation is well-known carcinogenic agent, however, the incidence of radiation-induced tumor is various from organ to organ, suggesting the tissue-type specific differences in the sensitivity to carcinogenic effects of radiation. Epidemiological studies including Atomic Bomb survivors and children around Chernobyl suggest that thyroid gland as well as bone marrow seem to be one of the most sensitive organs to the carcinogenic effects of external radiation (1,2). The accurate levels of radioactive iodine exposure to the thyroid glands remain to be further clarified among the children around Chernobyl (3,4), however, the vulnerable population is highly restricted in the group of the age between 0 to 5 year-old at the time of accident (5,6). The first joint program of Chernobyl Sasakawa project has been completed in 1996; among of which thyroid data are compiled and analyzed (7). To avoid the duplicated presentation, the summary of the past results has been briefly introduced at first (8). The reason why we have been working so intensively around Chernobyl is in part due to the necessity of improvement of the early diagnosis of thyroid diseases and overcome of the remoteness and inconvenience around Chernobyl. We have, therefore, introduced Telemedicine system to make a tight linkage and easy accessibility between Gomel and Nagasaki (9). So far early detection of childhood thyroid cancer has been successfully established using this system since February 1999. Until now more than 400 cases are consulted, among of whom, 12 cases of childhood thyroid cancer were diagnosed and surgically operated. To further extend this system, WHO-Sasakawa Health Telematics Project has also started, which includes Telepathology and Teleeducation between Minsk and Gomel, Belarus. (more detail information is available; http://www.who.int/pec/Radiation/healthtelepres.htm).

Moreover, the data management of the radiation-exposed victims is very much important.

Tissues from the thyroid tumors which are not needed for diagnostic purposes are valuable research resources, representing a large number of tumors directly related exposure to the same mutagen at the same time. The post-Chernobyl Thyroid Tissues, Nucleic Acids and Data Bank have been just established at the three countries (Minsk, Kiev and Obninsk) as an internationally supported cooperative research resource (further information website; http://www.wrl.cam.ac.uk/nisctb), which is now expected to avoid direct competition for limited tissue resources (10). Owing to such international collaboration, the infrastructure of scientific research on radiation-associated human thyroid carcinogenesis will be established.

1. The First Chernobyl Sasakawa Health and Medical Cooperation Project.

1.1. Subjects and methods

Territories radiocontaminated by the Chernobyl accident are vast, and, more than 4 million people resided in these contaminated areas. The subjects of study were children born between April 26, 1976 and April 26, 1986 (age at the time of accident: 0-10 years old), and examined in the period from May 15, 1991 to April 30, 1996. The data obtained from 120,000 children were analyzed and used for further evaluation. The course of health examination, either at the mobile diagnostic laboratory or at the center (Gomel and Mogilev in Belarus, Klincy in Russia, Kiev and Korosten in Ukraine), included the following; (1) collection of disease history and biographical information; (2) anthropometric data; (3) measurement of whole body Cs-137 radiation count; (4) ultrasonography of the thyroid; and (5) blood sampling for further analysis. Although we have all the health examination data, this presentation is focused on thyroid-related examination and the necessity of continuous screening and follow-up for these children will be discussed. The whole body Cs-137 counting data has been described elsewhere (11,12). Diagnosis of thyroid disease was established on the basis of the following criteria of thyroid images: (1) position, (2) structure, (3) echogenicity, (4) presence of nodules and cysts and (5) thyroid volume: The children were divided into two groups according to thyroid volume; normal and goiter. The criterion for goiter has been previously described (7).

The serum-free thyroid thyroxine (FT4) and thyroid stimulating hormone (TSH) levels were determined with Amerlite hormone analyzer. Titers of anti-thyroglobulin antibody (ATG) and anti-microsome antibody (AMC) were determined by the reaction of indirect hemagglutination (Fujirevio). Determination of iodine and creatinine content in the urine was carried out with a BRAN+LUBBE automatic Analyzer II (13). Four hundred and forty-six children showing echographic thyroid abnormalities were selected for fine-needle aspiration (FNA) biopsy, and a sample was successfully obtained for cytological diagnosis from 399 cases. Despite the presence of sampling bias of nodular lesions, cystic lesions and abnormal echo findings over 5mm in diameter, were chosen as targets for FNA. The diagnostic criteria for each disorder were described elsewhere (14,15).

1.2. Thyroid ultrasound

The eleven ultrasonograms taken from each subject (not just those with abnormal findings) are preserved semipermanently on optic disks. According to common diagnostic criteria, a prevalence of childhood goiter in the different distrincts of the five region has been described elsewhere (7). The incidence of goiter in the Mogilev region varied from 3 to 33% by district. The average goiter incidence was 22%. In contrast to the Mogilev region, there was a high prevalence of goiter in the Kiev region, Ukraine, with an average goiter incidence of 54%, which suggests that one of two children has an increased thyroid gland size. A large inter-regional variation was observed in the prevalence of goiter and it was highest in children from Kiev. A further investigation of geographical variation is needed in addition to the monitoring of iodide supplementation in school. The average frequency of thyroid nodules was 0.6%, and although FNB has not been performed in all cases, most of whom are thought to be either adenomatous goiter or adenoma. The highest incidence of thyroid nodule (1.64%) was observed in the Gomel region, Belarus. The frequency of abnormal echogenicity was also high in the Gomel region (4.09%), meanwhile Korosten was observed in the low frequency of abnormal echogenicity despite the high frequency of auto-antibody positive subjects.

1.3. Thyroid function

The results obtained, although within normal range (FT4, 10-25 pmol/l; TSH, 3-5mIU/ml) showed an uneven distribution. Based on the hormonal data and clinical findings, the incidence of thyroid dysfunction was also summarized (7), all of these patients need to be treated. The high incidence of hyperthyroidism in Mogilev region was thought to have been treated with an inappropriate medication of thyroid hormone (16). After excluding these artifacts, corrected incidence of hyperthyroidism in Mogilev region was 0.1% and there were no differences in the data among the five centers. Positive thyroid auto-antibody titers were found most frequently in Korosten (3%). The average among the five centers was 1.5% for ATG and 1.8% for AMC. Investigations are also being conducted to determine whether or not the frequency of auto-antibody-positive children in the Chernobyl region is reasonable on the basis of a comparison with other reports. The age-dependent increase of positive thyroid autoantibodies was also noticed, all of which data indicate the similar incidence of childhood chronic thyroiditis in the world. However, the increased incidence of juvenile hypothyroidism is suspected using our data analyzed with a group of Hanford downwinders (17).

1.4. FNA biopsy and cytological diagnosis

Cytological examinations were performed in 446 children, using echo-guided fine-needle aspiration (FNA) biopsy. The subjects were selected by the local staff, according to abnormal ultrasound findings in the thyroid. The percentage and distribution of the various diseases were demonstrated and 34 cases of childhood thyroid cancer were discovered. Other diseases, such as adenomatous goiter, cyst and chronic thyroiditis, were also confirmed by cytology or in combination with other laboratory data. A high incidence of cancer was observed in Gomel, which was supported by the evidence that the prevalence of thyroid nodules and abnormal echogenicity findings in this area. Among 446 subjects by FNA cytological diagnosis with ultrasonographic findings, most cases of papillary carcinoma and follicular neoplasm were found in subjects showing nodular pattern and hypoechogenic changes by ultrasonography, while chronic thyroiditis was detected mainly in subjects showing abnormal echogenicity. The malignant cases suspected by FNA cytology were all confirmed by surgical histology at the Misnk Thyroid Oncology Center (18). From 1996 to 2000, more than 20 cases of childhood thyroid cancer have been detected within the second Chernobyl Sasakawa Project, which data are now under analysis.

1.5. Urinary iodine concentration

As the incidence of goiter differed widely in the Mogilev and Kiev regions, urinary iodine secretion was measured in some children in the different districts. In Mogilev, about 20% of children had less than 10mg/dl urinary iodine, where the deficiency was not correctly compensated by iodine supplementation. These results support the evidence of different degrees of endemic goiter around Chernobyl (19). As a result, there were 40 groups consisting of 5652 children around Chernobyl, a significant negative correlation was observed between the prevalence of goiter and the median level of urinary iodine excretion. Although there are two centers; Mogilev and Kiev, for measurement of urinary iodine, routine activities are stopped.

Now we have introduced a novel type of equipment of urinary iodine measurement to the Endocrinology Institute in Moscow to further extend our cooperative project.

2. The Second Chernobyl Sasakawa Health Cooperation Project

Since the high incidence of childhood thyroid diseases has been demonstrated around Chernobyl, especially in Gomel region, Belarus, we have further continued several medical aid projects, focusing on the early diagnosis and careful follow-up for children who have been detected thyroid abnormalities by ultrasound examination. Simultaneously we used an epidemiological approach to elucidate the cause-and-effect relationship between Chernobyl accident, especially short-lived radionuletides, and childhood thyroid cancer. The application of comparative study is now under investigation in children who were born before and after the accident in Gomel region. The target population number is 30,000. Our preliminary data suggest that there is no childhood thyroid cancer who were born after the accident. According to the Belarussian National Tumor Registry, however, sixteen cases of operated childhood thyroid cancer who were born after the accident and in Ukraine, nineteen cases, were reported, respectively.

The joint project with International Agency for Research on Cancer (IARC) is also under analysis, which involves operated childhood thyroid cancer patients in Gomel and partly in Mogilev., respectively. The target number of case-control study is about 250 patients and 1500 controls. In Russia, same case-control study has been completed and now under analysis. The unique cohort study has been conducted in Kaluga, Oreol and Tula regions in Russian Federation, in cooperation with Medical Radiological Research Center, RAMS, Obninsk. Furthermore there are relatively highly exposed population in the western region of Bryansk (20). All these studies are now under investigation and so any data cannot be presented here so far.

However, it is important how to analyze these data and utilize such invaluable materials for future studies. Concerning the operated childhood thyroid cancer tissues, it would be worthy to analyze the signature genes or proteins induced by radiation-exposure. Indeed gene rearrangements of ret/PTC subtypes have been reported as a common genetic damage of radiation-induced thyroid cancer (21,22). Unfortunately, there is no specific and selective marker to identify the radiation-induced signature genes. Therefore now Chernobyl Thyroid Tissue Bank has just started to promote the scientific cooperation internationally (10).

3. Radiation-induced thyroid carcinogenesis

3.1. Influence to thyroid cell membrane by radiation

Based on the above Chernobyl Sasakawa Humanitarian Medical Aid Projects, it is urgent to clarify the cause-and-effect relationship between the Chernobyl accident and any health consequence, especially childhood thyroid cancer. To understand the molecular mechanism of radiation-induced thyroid carcinogenesis, we must at first realize that human thyroid cells are relatively resistant to apoptosis caused by ionizing radiation (23, 24), although the latter can cause both DNA damage and cell membrane breakdown (25,26). Our experimental results have demonstrated that the radioresistant properties of human thyroid cells is in part due to the dominance of anti-apoptotic signals evoked by growth factors and diacylglycerol, which override the apoptotic effect of ceramide released from human thyroid cell membrane on exposure of ionizing radiation (27). Furthermore the downstream target molecules, such as c-JUN N-terminal kinase (JNK) phosphorylation pattern, are unique in human thyroid cells, which may be involved in cell survival, not in apoptosis (28). An improved understanding of JNK-mediated apoptotic signaling may provide novel strategies in prevention and treatment of cancers (29). The reason why we need to pay special attention to such cell survival and escape mechanism from apoptosis is that low-dose irradiation can cause abnormal cell proliferation through constitutive activation of intracellular target molecules and disturb the apoptosis-prone pathways, besides the direct genetic alteration (Fig. 1). JNK activation by irradiation may contribute to cell survival. Furthermore the involvement of cell cycle checkpoint pathway should be further analyzed at the standpoint of radiosensitivity and radioresistancy (30). Unique response of thyroid cells, especially intracellular signal transduction system, may contribute to abnormal cell proliferation after low-dose irradiation.

3.2. DNA damages by radiation

It is obvious, however, that a high prevalence of ret rearrangements (62.3%) with a significant predominance of ELE1/ret (PTC3) over H4/ret (PTC1) rearrangement was found in childhood papillary thyroid carcinomas of the first Chernobyl decade (31). Furthermore low frequency of other types of gene rearrangements (32) and absence of point mutations (33) have been also reported. Therefore, attention has been focused on the direct relationship between the rapid increase of childhood thyroid cancer and ret/PTC gene rearrangements, implicating the characteristics of post-Chernobyl thyroid cancers; biological, phenotypical and clinical from genetic alternation (34). In contrast, the role and significant of ret/PTC may be far away from our current understanding because of high frequency of these rearrangement observed in papillary thyroid carcinoma in New Caledonia and Australia (35). The age-related ret/PTC rearrangement should be, therefore, analyzed (Table 1)

To further understand the molecular genetic aberrations and microsatellite instabilities (36), careful and advanced analysis has been undergone using the modern molecular biology techniques.

At the standpoint of basic medical research, therefore, any clinical data and biomaterials should be kept, managed and used for future sophisticated analysis.

4. Conclusion

There is no substantive proof regarding radiation-induced teratogenic effects from the Chernobyl accident (37), however, only childhood thyroid carcinoma is strongly considered to be directly related to short-lived radioiodines massively released just after the accident to the vast territories around Chernobyl. The challenge for retrospective reconstruction of thyroid dose for inhabitants around Chernobyl has been intensively continued (38, 39). The late effect of radiation, even in the lower dose, on human thyroid glands should be monitored carefully for the radiation-sensitive vulnerable group around Chernobyl for a longer period and the direct signature gene(s) by radiation-induced thyroid cancer should be clarified through investigation of advanced molecular biology techniques. Chernobyl Sasakawa Medical Cooperation Project is, therefore, not only a unique humanitarian-aid but also the most serious scientific program with worldwide implications. The continuation of this program is now strongly recommended and desired. Alternatively smooth succession of medical aid programs is essential and expected from the international societies as well as from three counties; Belarus, Russia and Ukraine.

Reference

1. Ron E, Lubin JH, Shore RE et al (1995) Thyroid cancer after exposure to external radiation: a pooled analysis of seven studies. Radiation Res 141; 259-277
2. United Nations Scientific Committee on the Effects of Atomic Radiation. Sources and effects of ionizing radiation. UNSCARE 2000 Report to the General Assembyl, with scientific annexes. New York, United Nations, 2000
3. Bleuer JP, Averkin YI, Abelin T (1997) Chernobyl-related thyroid cancer: what evidence for role of short-lived iodines? Environ Health Perspect 6:1483-1486
4. Goulko GM, Chepurny NI, Jacob P, Kairo IA, Likhtarev IA, Prohl G, Sobolev BG (1998) Thyroid dose and thyroid cancer incidence after the Chernobyl accident: assesments for the Zhytomyr region, Ukraine. Radiat Environ Biophys. 36:261-273
5. Pacini F, Vorontsova T, Demidchik EP et al (1997) Post-Chernobyl thyroid carcinoma in Belarus children and adolescence: comparison with naturally occurring thyroid carcinoma in Italy and France. J Clin Endocrinol Metab. 82:3563-3569
6. Farahati J, Demidchik EP, Biko J, Reiner C (2000) Inverse association between age at the time of radiation exposure and extension of disease in cases of radiation-induced thyroid carcinomas in Belarus. Cancer. 88:1470-14476

7.   Yamashita S, Shibata S (1997) Chernobyl: A Decade, Excerta Medica, Amsterdam, ICS 1156, pp613

8.   Yamasihta S, Ito M, Ashizawa K, Shibata Y, Nagataki S, Kiikuni K (1999) Monitoring and prevention of the development of thyroid carcinoma in a population exposed to radiation. Radiation and Thyroid Cancer eds by Thomas G, Karaoglou A, Williams ED. World Scientific, 369-376

9.   Yamashita S, Shibata Y, Takamura N et al (1999) Satellite Communication and Medical Assistance for Thyroid Disease Diagnosis from Nagasaki to Chernobyl. Thyroid 9: 969

10.   Thomas GA, Williams ED and Members of the Scientific Project Panel (2000) Thyroid tumor bank. Science 289:2283

11.   Hoshi M, Yamamoto M, Kawamura H et al (1994) Fallout radioactivity in soil and food samples in the Ukraine: measurement of iodine, plutonium, cesium and strontium isotopes. Health Phys 67: 187-191

12.   Hoshi M, Shibata Y, Okajima S et al (1994) Cesium-137 concentration among children in areas contaminated with radioactive fallout caused by the Chernobyl accident; the results in Gomel and Mogilev oblasts, Belarus. Health Phys 67: 268-271

13.   Tsuda K, Namba H, Nomura T et al (1995) Automated measurement of urinary iodine with use of ultraviolet irradiation. Clin Chem 414: 581-585

14.   Ito M, Yamashita S, Ashizawa K et al (1995) Childhood thyroid disease around Chernobyl evaluated by fine needle aspiration cytology. Thyroid 5: 365-368

15.   Ito M, Kotova L, Panasyuk G et al (1997) Cytological characteristics of pediatric thyroid cancer around Chernobyl. Act Cytol 41: 1642-1644

16.   Ashizawa K, Krupnik T, Nagataki S, Yamashita S (1998) Transient thyrotoxicosis around Chernobyl. Thyroid 8: 535-536

17.   Glodsmith JR, Grossman CM, Morton WE et al (1999) Juvenile hypothyoidism among two populations exposed to radioiodine. Environ Health Perspect 107: 303-308

18.   Ito M, Yamashita S, Ashizawa K et al (1996) Histopathological characteristics of childhood thyroid cancer in Gomel, Belarus. International J Cancer 65: 29-33

19.   Ashizawa K, Shibata Y, Yamashita S et al (1997) Prevalence of goiter and urinary iodine excretion levels in children around Chernobyl. J Clin Endocrinol Metab 82: 3430-3433

20.   Hoshi M, Konstantinov YO, Evdeeva TY et al (2000) Radio-cesium in children residing in the western districs of the Bryansk oblast from 1991-1996. Health Physics 79: 182-186

21.   Tuttle RM, Becker DV (2000) The Chernobyl accident ant its consequences: update at the millennium. Semin Nucl Med 30: 133-140

22.   Nikiforva MN, Stringer JR, Blogh R, Medvedovic M, Fagin JA, Nikiforv YE (2000) Proximity of chromosomal loci that participate in radiation-induced rearrangements in human cells. Science 290: 138-141

23.   Namba H, Hara T, Tsukazaki T et al (1995) Radiation-induced G1 arrest is selectively mediated by the p53-WAF1/Cip1 pathway in human thyroid cells. Cancer Res 55: 2075-2080

24.   Yang T, Namba H, Hara T et al (1997) p53 induced by ionizing radiation medicates DNA end-joining activity, but not apoptosis of thyroid cells. Oncogene 14: 1511-1519

25.   Dugle DL, Gillespie CJ, Chapman JD (1976) DNA strand breaks, repair and survival in X-irradiated mammalian cells. Proc Natl Acad Sci, USA. 73:809-812

26.   Canman CE, Lim DS, Cimprich KA et al (1998) Activation of the ATM kinase by ionizing radiation and phosphorylation of p53. Science 281: 1677-1679

27.   Sautin Y, Takamura N, Shkylaev S et al (2000) Ceramide-induced apoptosis of human thyroid cancer cells resistant to apoptosis by irradiation. Thyroid 10:733-740

28.   Shklyaev S, Namba H, Mitsutake N et al (2000) Transient activation of c-Jun NH2-terminal kinase by growth factors influences survival but not apoptosis in human thyrocytes. (in press) Thyroid

29.   Chen YR, Tan TH (2000) The c-Jun N-terminal kinase pathway and apoptotic signaling. International J Oncol. 16:651-662

30.   Falck J, Mailand N, Syljuasen RG, Bartek J, Lukas J (2001) The AMT-Chk2-Cdc25A checkpoint pathway guards against radioresistant DNA synthesis. Nature 410:842-847

31.   Rabes HM, Klugbauer S (1998) Molecular genetics of child-hood papillary thyroid carcinomas after irradiation: high prevalence of RET rearrargement. Recent Results Cancer Res 154: 248-264

32. Beimfohr C, Klumbauer S, Demidchik, Lengfelder E, Rabes HM (1999) NTRK1 rearrangemnet in papillary thyroid carcinomas of children after the Chernobyl reactor accident. Int J Cancer 80: 842-847

33. Suchy B, Waldmann V, Klugbauer S, Rabes HM (1998) Absence of RAS and p53 mutations in htyrpoid carcinomas of children after the Chernobyl in contarst to adult thyroid tumors. Br J Cancer 77: 952-955

34. Rabes HM, Demidchik EP, Sidorov JD et al (2000) Pattern of radiation-induced RET and NTRK1 rearrangements in 191 post-Chernobyl papillary thyroid carcinomas: biological, phenotypic and clinical implications. Clin Cancer Res 6: 10930-1103

35. Chua EL, Wu WM, Tran KT et al (2000) Prevalence and distribution of ret/ptc 1,2 and 3 in papillary thyroid carcinoma in New Caledonia and Australia. J Clin Endocrinol Metab 85: 2733-2739

36. Richter H, Lohrer HD, Hieber L et al (1999) Microsatellite instability and loss of heterozygosity in radiation-associated thyroid carcinomas of Belarussian children and adults. Carcinogenesis 20: 2247-2252

37. Casronovo FP (1999) Teratogen update: radiation and Chernobyl. Teratology 60: 100-106

38. Straume T, Annspaugh LR, Haskell EH et al (1997) Emerging echnological bases for retrospective dosimetry. Stem Cells 15: 83-93

39. Gavrilin YI, Khrouch VT, Shinkarev SM et al (1999) Chernobyl accident: reconstruction of thyroid dose for inhabitants of the Republic of Belarus. 76: 105-119

40. Mitsutake N, Namba H, Shklyaev SS et al (2001) PKC delta mediates ionizing radiation-induced activation of c-Jun NH2 terminal kinase through MKK7 in human thyroid cells. Oncogene 20: 989-996

Acknowledgment

This review was supported in part by grants-in-aid for scientific research from the Japanese Ministry of Education, Science, Sports and Culture (No.12470221, No.12576020).

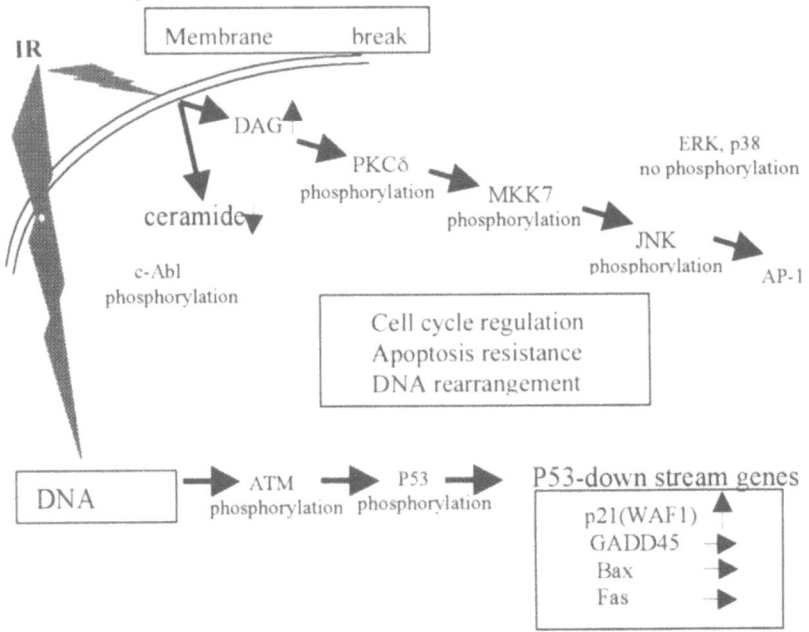

Fig. 1. Schema of the effect of low-dose radiation and thyroid cell response. The mechanism of radiation-induced intracellular signal transduction activation is summarized based on our own data. In response to radiation-exposure, thyroid cell membrane breakdown occurs and selectively increased level of diacylgylcerol (DAG) stimulates PKC delta phosphorylation, which cascade works through MKK7 and Jun phosphorylation activation, then finally reaches to AP1 activation (40), resulting in the predominant characteristic of cell survival. Besides the direct damage of double stranded DNA breaks, downstream target molecules, p53 and p21 are selectively activated and the disturbance of cell cycle is induced such as cell cycle arrest. The cell survival stimulation by low-dose irradiation may also influence the resistance to cell apoptosis. Such abnormal cell survival mechanism may result in high incidence of ret/PTC gene rearrangement, especially in childhood thyroid glands after irradiation.

Table 1. The incidence of ret/PTC rearrangement reported by various papers in adult cases (upper) and in children (lower). References are as follows;

Wajjwalku W et al; Jpn J Cancer Res. 1992,83;671, Ishizaka Y et al; Oncogene. 1989,4;789, Namba H et al; Endocrinol Jpn. 1991, 38;627, Motomura et al; Thyroid. 1998, 8;485, Bongarzone I et al; Oncogene. 1989, 4;1457, Cancer Res. 1994, 5429;79 and J Clin Endocrinol Metab 1996, 81;2006, .Santoro M et al; J Clin Invest. 1992, 89;1517, Jhiang SM et al; Oncogene. 1992, 7;1331, Sugg SL et al; J Clin Endocrinol Metab, 1996, 81;3360, Zou M et al; Cancer. 1994, 73;176,, Mayr B et al; Br J Cancer 1998, 77;903, Lee CH et al; J Clin Endocrinol Metab 1998, 83;1629, Chua EL et al; J Clin Endocrinol Metab 2000, 85;2753, Nikiforov YE et al; Cancer Res 1997, 57;1690, Klugbauer S at al; Oncogene. 1995, 11;2459, Fugazzola L et al; Oncogene 1996, 13; 1093

Country	Reference	Ret/PTC	Method
Japan	Wajjiwalku	3% (1/38)	RT-PCR
	Ishizawa	9% (111)	RT-PCR
	Namba	0% (0/10)	RT-PCR
	Nishikawa	36% (4/11)	Southern / RT-PCR
Italy	Bongarzone	35% (18/52)	Focus assay Southern / RT-PCR
USA	Santoro	17% (11/65)	Southern / RT-PCR
	Jhiang	11% (4/36)	Southern / RT-PCR
France	Santoro	11% (8/70)	RT-PCR
Canada	Sugg	5.3% (3/57)	RT-PCR
Saudi Arabia	Zou	2.5% (1/40)	RT-PCR
Germany	Mayr	8% (8/99)	RT-PCR
Taiwan	Lee	55% (6/11)	RT-PCR
Australia	Chua	85% (17/20)	Southern / RT-PCR
New Caledonia	Chua	70% (19/27)	Southern / RT-PCR

(Adult)

Country	Reference	Ret/PTC	Method
Japan	Nishikawa	30% (3/10)	Southern / RT-PCR
Italy	Bongarzone	67% (6/9)	Southern / RT-PCR
USA	Nikiforov	71% (12/17)	Southern / RT-PCR
Belarus	Klugbauer	67% (8/12)	RT-PCR
	Fugazzola	67% (4/6)	Focus assay Southern / RT-PCR
	Nikiforov	87% (33/38)	RT-PCR

(Children)

GENETIC EVENTS IN RADIATION-INDUCED THYROID CANCER

Yuri E. Nikiforov, M.D., Ph.D.
Department of Pathology, University of Cincinnati, USA.

Key Words
thyroid neoplasms, ionizing radiation, radioiodines, radiation-induced thyroid cancer, post-Chernobylm, *RAS, p53, RET,* PTC, *RET*/PTC

Exposure to ionizing radiation is a well-established risk factor for a number of human solid neoplasms and hematologic malignancies. Among them, thyroid cancer is a striking example of tumors that have a well-documented association with both medical/therapeutic and accidental environmental types of radiation exposure. Here, I would like to review what we have learned over the last decade about the genetic events associated with radiation-induced carcinogenesis in the thyroid gland.

The association between radiation to the thyroid gland area and thyroid cancer was first proposed in 1950 in children who received X-ray therapy in infancy for an enlarged thymus (1). During the following decades, numerous reports have documented an increased incidence of thyroid neoplasms in patients after external radiation for different benign conditions of the head, neck and thorax (2). Since 1965, when the use of radiotherapy for benign conditions was abandoned, the incidence of radiation-associated thyroid malignancy gradually decreased (3). Currently, radiation therapy for malignancy continues to be a source of radiation-associated thyroid cancer. The increased risk of thyroid cancer was also linked to environmental irradiation. This was documented in survivors exposed to gamma and neutron radiation after the atomic bomb explosions in Japan in 1945 (4), and in residents of the Marshall Islands exposed to fallout after detonation of a thermonuclear device on the Bikini atoll in 1954, where thyroid exposure resulted from internal irradiation due to absorption of radioiodines and penetrating gamma radiation (5). In the U.S., exposure to radioiodines from atmospheric nuclear tests in Nevada in the 1950s was linked to an excess of thyroid neoplasms, and a dose response was suggested for children under 1 year of age at exposure (6,7).

The long-term follow-up of populations subjected to therapeutic or environmental irradiation allowed characterization of epidemiological and clinical features of radiation-induced thyroid cancer (8-10). Thyroid cancers begin to develop 5-10 years after exposure, reach a maximum incidence in 25-29 years, and in most cases the relative risk remains elevated after 40-45 years. There is strong inverse correlation with age at exposure and a linear dose response in a wide range of the absorbed doses. Papillary carcinoma is the predominant type of thyroid cancer, and overall prognosis of radiation-induced papillary carcinomas is comparable to that of sporadic tumors.

Thus, the association between radiation and thyroid cancer has a firm clinical/epidemiological basis. However, until recently, little progress was made in our understanding of the molecular mechanisms underlying radiation carcinogenesis in the thyroid gland. This can be explained in part by unavailability of current molecular biology tools, and by the fact that pediatric and adult populations followed for several decades after exposure were in time "diluted" by a large number of sporadic thyroid tumors, the incidence of which rises considerably in individuals after the age of 20 years.

Over the last decade, an interest to this topic was reborn because of the accident at the Chernobyl Nuclear Power Station in the former USSR in April 1986. This tragic accident produced one of the most serious environmental disasters ever recorded and led to a dramatic increase in the frequency of childhood thyroid cancer in contaminated areas of Belarus, Ukraine, and western regions of Russia (11-12). Because of the extremely low incidence of sporadic thyroid carcinoma in children before the accident, as well as in those born after 1986 (12), it can be assumed that almost all pediatric thyroid tumors from the affected areas are associated with exposure to radiation. Thus, this tragic disaster created one of the richest paradigms of radiation-induced human neoplasia, offering a unique opportunity to examine the molecular mechanisms of radiation-induced thyroid cancer.

Histologically, more than 90% of post-Chernobyl thyroid cancers were papillary carcinomas (13). A distinguishing feature of these tumors was the high prevalence of a solid growth pattern, which appeared as sheets of malignant epithelial cells surrounded by varying amounts of fibrotic stroma (Fig. 1). Thus, in a series of 84 cases operated in Belarus in 1991-1992, the solid growth pattern was seen in almost half of all Chernobyl cancers, including 34% of tumors containing exclusively or predominantly of solid areas and another 12% of cases which contained solid areas admixed with follicular and/or papillary components (14). Similar data were obtained in a larger series of post-Chernobyl tumors from Belarus and Ukraine, where more than 50% of papillary carcinomas were of solid-follicular type (15). By contrast, this type of growth is rare in spontaneous adult and pediatric papillary carcinomas that show predominantly classical papillary growth. This, only 4% of papillary carcinomas in children with no history of radiation exposure from two different regions in the U.S. were the solid variants (16).

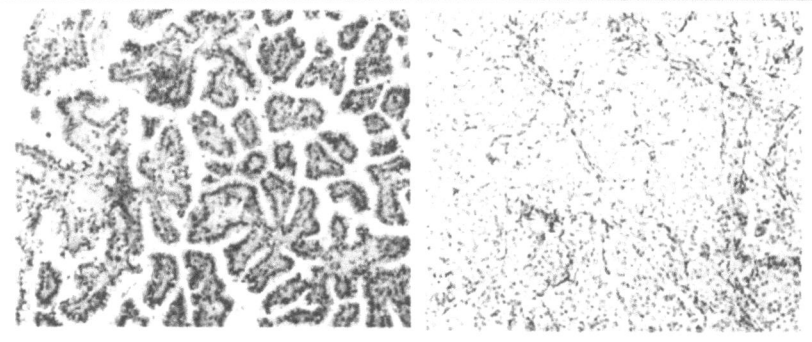

Fig. 1. Microscopic appearance of classical papillary thyroid cancer most prevalent in sporadic populations (left) and of the solid variant of papillary carcinoma which is common in post-Chernobyl populations (right).

The initial studies of radiation-induced thyroid tumors have focused on the genes known to be mutated in the sporadic forms of the disease. One of the first candidates to be explored was the proto-oncogene *RAS*, a membrane-associated protein that transmits signals arising after ligand binding to tyrosine kinase receptors. Point mutations of the three *RAS* genes are reported in 18-62% of papillary thyroid carcinoma, and with even greater prevalence in follicular thyroid tumors (reviewed in (17)). It has been suggested that *K-RAS* mutations may be associated with radiation exposure, since they constituted 3 out of 4 (75%) *RAS* mutations in a group of patient with a history of therapeutic external radiation, whereas only 6 out of 25 (25%) mutation in a control group of sporadic tumors were *K-RAS* (18). However, in should be noted that most of these cases were follicular neoplasms rather than papillary carcinomas. In another study, *RAS* mutations were found in 30% of thyroid tumors from patients with a history of external irradiation and in 42% of sporadic thyroid tumors, and similar prevalence of *K-RAS* mutations was observed in both groups (19). We analyzed the prevalence of *RAS* mutation in a series of 33 post-Chernobyl papillary carcinomas, one follicular carcinoma, and 22 benign nodular lesions from Belarus (20). No *RAS* mutations was detected in papillary carcinomas, whereas 1/1 case of follicular carcinoma and 3/7 follicular adenomas were positive for *N-RAS* codon 61 mutations. Only 2 *RAS* mutations were found in another series of 44 post-Chernobyl papillary carcinomas, and none of them were in critical codons 12, 13, or 61 (21). The absence of *RAS* mutations in papillary carcinomas was also observed in the study by Santoro et al. who analyzed 31 post-Chernobyl tumors for K-*RAS* mutations and 23 for *N-RAS* and *H-RAS* mutations (22). It is conceivable that radiation may induce at least two distinct pathways of tumor initiation, and that *RAS* activation through point mutations may predispose to formation of follicular neoplasms. However, point mutations of the *RAS* gene do not play a significant role in the development of papillary carcinomas after radiation exposure (Table 1).

Table 1. *Prevalence of RAS Mutations in Radiation-Induced Thyroid Tumors*

Therapeutic Radiation	
Wright et al. (1991)[18]	4/12 (33%) after radiation, 3/4 *K-RAS* in follicular carcinomas
	25/68 (37%) in non-radiation group, 6/25 *K- RAS*
Challeton et al. (1995)[19]	10/33 (30%) after radiation
	36/86 (42%) spontaneous, similar prevalence of *K- RAS* mutations
Environmental Radiation	*(Post-Chernobyl Tumors)*
Nikiforov et al. (1996)[20]	0/33 in papillary carcinomas
	3/7 in follicular adenomas
	1/1 in follicular carcinoma
Suchy et al. (1998)[21]	2/44 in papillary carcinomas (none in codons 12, 13, or 61)
Santoro et al. (2000)[22]	0/23 in papillary carcinomas

Point mutations of the *p53* tumor suppressor gene have also been studied in radiation-induced thyroid tumors. The *p53* protein is involved in the cell cycle regulation, largely by its ability to transactivate expression of genes coding for proteins such as p21/WAF1 that induce G_1 arrest. In addition, *p53* can help trigger a program of apoptosis. Inactivating point mutations of the *p53* tumor suppressor gene are highly prevalent in anaplastic and poorly-differentiated thyroid tumors, but not in well-differentiated papillary or follicular carcinomas (reviewed in (17)). However, as discussed above, thyroid papillary carcinomas in children after Chernobyl are characterized by a high prevalence of solid growth that considered by some authors as evidence of a more malignant phenotype.

Missense point mutations in exons 5-8 of the *p53* gene have been found in 4 out of 22 (18%) papillary carcinomas developed in patients exposed in childhood to radiation in the head and neck area (23). Several studies reported the prevalence of *p53* mutations in post-Chernobyl tumors. Utilizing PCR-SSCP analysis, we studied 33 post-Chernobyl papillary carcinomas for point mutations in exons 5-8 of *p53* and observed two (6%) somatic mutations, both in exon 5 (20). Sequence analysis that showed one of those mutations to be a missense mutation and another to be a silent mutation. A slightly higher prevalence of *p53* mutations was observed by Hillebrandt et al. who studied mutations in exons 4-9 of *p53* by PCR-TGGE (24). They found 6 (23%) mutations in exons 6 and 7 which were not further characterized by sequencing. In another study, a 16% prevalence of *p53* mutations was reported among 31 pediatric papillary carcinomas from Belarus, all were in codon 213 of exon 6 (25). Recently, Santoro et al. reported no exon 5-8 *p53* mutations in a series of 35 post-Chernobyl tumors (22). Although the prevalence of p53 mutations in these studies was somewhat variable, the overall prevalence was still low. A metanalysis of all these post-Chernobyl studies shows a 10% prevalence of *p53* mutations (Table 2). This indicates that inactivation of this tumor suppressor gene may play only a limited role in radiation-induced papillary thyroid carcinoma formation.

Therapeutic radiation	
Fogelfeld et al. (1996)[23]	4/22 (18%) after radiation
	0/18 PTC in control group
Environmental Radiation (post-Chernobyl tumors)	
Hillebrandt et al. (1996)[24]	6/26 (23%)
Nikiforov et al. (1996)[20]	2/33 (6%)
Smida et al. (1997)[25]	5/31 (16%)
Santoro et al. (2000)[22]	0/35
Total post-Chernobyl:	13/125 (10%)

Mutations of TSH receptor gene and *GSP* mutations were also studied in radiation-induced thyroid tumors, and the absence or low prevalence of these mutations was found in tumors associated with external radiation (19) and in post-Chernobyl tumors (22,26).

In addition to point mutations, a number of other genetic events have been studied in radiation-induced thyroid tumors. One of such events was a genomic instability. The hypothesis of genome destabilization after radiation exposure was attractive, especially in the light of a study reporting a higher rate of germline mutations at human hypervariable minisatellite loci in children born from parents exposed to radiation after Chernobyl (27). The prevalence of two forms of genome destabilization, somatic minisatellite and microsatellite instability, was tested in post-Chernobyl papillary thyroid carcinomas. Although several mutations in minisatellite and microsatellite loci was found, the overall prevalence of either type of instability was low (28,29). Loss of heterozygosity (LOH) was seen in very few loci in 6% (28) and 25% (29) of post-Chernobyl papillary carcinomas. These data suggest that overall there is no significant genome destabilization in papillary thyroid carcinomas arising after radiation exposure. This also suggested that discrete mutation events should be important for tumor development after radiation exposure.

It is clear today that at least one of such important genetic abnormalities is a rearrangement of the *RET* proto-oncogene. The *RET* gene, located on chromosome 10q11.2, encodes a transmembrane receptor with a tyrosine kinase activity (30). Its ligand has been recently identified as neurotrophic factors of the glial cell-line derived neurotrophic factor

(GDNF) family, including GDNF, neurturin, artemin, and persephin. Since the original report of *RET* activation through rearrangement in papillary thyroid carcinomas (31), three major types of this chimeric gene have been identified (Fig. 2). All are derived from the fusion of the tyrosine kinase domain of *RET* with 5'-regions of different genes. Two of these types, *RET*/PTC1 and *RET*/PTC3, are the results of an intrachromosomal rearrangement. *RET* /PTC1 is formed by fusion of *RET* with a gene named *H4*/D10S170 (31), and *RET*/PTC3 is a product of *RET* fusion with the *ELE1* gene (32,33). *RET*/PTC2 is formed by a reciprocal translocation between chromosomes 10 and 17, resulting in fusion with the 5' terminal sequence of the regulatory subunit of *RIα* cAMP-dependent PKA (34). The genes that become illegitimately coupled to the *RET* tyrosine kinase domain are expressed ubiquitously, and drive the expression of the truncated *RET* receptor in thyroid follicular cells. Recently, a number of single cases of other types of *RET*/PTC rearrangement were described, where fragments of other genes were fused with the tyrosine kinase domain of *RET* (reviewed in (35)).

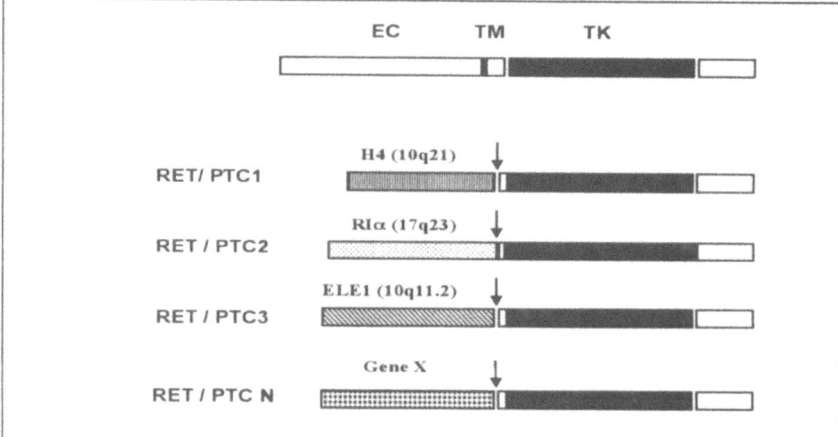

Fig. 2. *Schematic representation of the wild-type RET gene and activated forms of RET/PTC rearrangements in human papillary thyroid carcinomas. (EC - extracellular domain, TM - transemembrane domain, TK- tyrosine kinase domain of RET)*

RET/PTC rearrangements have been reported in 2.5-34% of sporadic papillary carcinomas in the general (mostly adult) populations. Among them, *RET*/PTC1 is by far the most common type, comprising approximately 70% of all *RET*/PTC rearrangements, *RET*/PTC3 is seen in 10-30% of cases, and *RET*/PTC 2 in less than 10%.

A much higher prevalence of *RET*/PTC has been observed in post-Chernobyl pediatric papillary carcinomas. The first reports of tumors removed 5-8 years after the accident demonstrated *RET* rearrangements in 67%-87% of cases, and two-thirds of them were of the *RET*/PTC3 type (36-37). In our series of 38 post-Chernobyl papillary carcinomas from 1991-1992, 87% of tumors showed evidence of *RET* rearrangements (16). Among them, 67% of tumors were positive for *RET*/PTC3 and 18% for *RET*/PTC1. The high prevalence of *RET*/PTC rearrangements and predominance of the *RET*/PTC3 type have been observed in other series (Table 3).

Table 3. *Prevalence of RET/PTC Rearrangements in Radiation-Induced Thyroid Cancer Total RET/PTC1   RET/PTC2   RET/PTC3 RET/PTC*

	Total		RET/PTC1	RET/PTC2	RET/PTC3
Environmental Radiation (post-Chernobyl)					
Ito et al. (1994)[3]	4/7	(57%)	?	?	?
Klugbauer et al. (1995)[36]	8/12	(67%)	17%	0	50%
Fugazzola et al. (1995)[37]	4/6	(67%)	0	16%	50%
Nikiforov et al. (1997)[16]	33/38	(87%)	16%	3%	58%
Smida et al. (1999)[39]	32/51	(63%)	24%	0	26%
Rabes et al.(2000)[40]	94/191	(49%)	25%	0	20%
External Therapeutic Radiation					
Bounacer et al (1997)[41]	16/19	(84%)	74%	0	21%

A significant correlation between different types of *RET*/PTC and morphological variants of papillary carcinoma has been found. Thus, we observed that the solid variant of papillary carcinoma correlates with *RET*/PTC3, and typical papillary pattern of tumor with *RET*/PTC1 type of rearrangement (16). Such correlation was confirmed in a series of post-Chernobyl tumors from Belarus and Ukraine from 1990-1995 (15) and in mouse transgenic models. Thus, thyroid-specific expression of the *RET*/PTC1 chimeric gene under the control of the rat (42) or bovine (43) thyroglobulin promoter resulted in development of slowly progressing thyroid papillary carcinomas with papillary or mixed architecture, whereas transgenic mice expressing *RET*/PTC3 chimeric gene under the control of the bovine thyroglobulin promoter developed thyroid tumors with a solid histological phenotype (44).

As for post-Chernobyl tumors removed after a longer latency period, they also showed a high prevalence of *RET* rearrangements, but *RET*/PTC1 was the most common type (Table 4) (39,40). This may suggest that tumors initiated by *RET*/PTC3 have a higher growth rate than those with *RET*/PTC1. This is supported by the fact that *RET*/PTC3 transgenic mice demonstrate more malignant phenotype and metastatic disease as compared to *RET*/PTC1 animals (44).

Table 4. *RET/PTC Prevalence After Chernobyl: Correlation With the Latency Period (40)*

Latency perio	Total	RET/PTC1	RET/PTC3
≤10 years	40/61 (66%)	23%	60%
> 10 years	60/130 (46%)	65%	23%

These data indicate that rearrangements of the *RET* gene are the major genetic event in a well-characterized population of radiation-induced post-Chernobyl papillary carcinomas. In addition, *RET* rearrangements were found in 84% of papillary carcinomas from patients who had received external radiation (41). *RET*/PTC1 rearrangements can be also induced by irradiation of human undifferentiated thyroid carcinoma cells in-vitro (45) and of fetal human thyroid tissue transplanted to SCID mice (46). In both observations, *RET*/PTC1 was detected by RT-PCR as soon as 2 days after exposure. The effective dose of radiation in both of these studies was high (50 Gy), and the cells used in the initial report were already highly transformed, and hence more susceptible to develop secondary genetic defects. Nevertheless, these observations demonstrate that radiation can directly induce *RET*/PTC rearrangements. All these suggest that *RET*/PTC rearrangements have direct association with radiation exposure, and unraveling mechanisms of its generation after radiation exposure is crucial to the understanding of radiation-induced carcinogenesis in the thyroid gland.

There are two most possible pathways of *RET*/PTC generation after radiation exposure: direct, when *RET*/PTC is an immediate result of double-strand DNA breaks produced by radiation, and indirect, when the re-arrangement occurs later, after all DNA breaks are repaired. Significant information in this regard has been obtained by mapping the exact breakpoint sites in the *RET* and *ELE1* genes in 12 post-Chernobyl tumors with *RET*/PTC3 rearrangement (47). The breakpoint cluster regions in these gene reside are known to be within *ELE1* intron 5 (1670 bp) and *RET* intron 11 (1843bp) (48). If the *RET*/PTC arose late in tumor progression as a result of activation or disruption of the recombination machinery, one would expect the breaks to be located within recombinase signal sequences at both participating loci, to have similarity in sequences at the breakpoints, and to be clustered at certain specific hypersensitive DNA regions. By contrast, we found that in post-Chernobyl tumors the *RET*/PTC breakpoints were distributed randomly across the respective introns, except for some clustering in the Alu repeats of one of the two contributing genes, with no breakpoints occurring at exactly the same base or within an identical sequence in any of the 12 tumors (Fig. 3) (47). The breakpoints exhibited no particular nucleotide sequence or composition. Thus, there was no evidence of consistency in AT-rich regions, fragile sites, recombination-specific signal elements, or other target DNA sites (i.e. *chi*-like motifs, heptamer/nonamer signal sequences) implicated in illegitimate recombination in mammalian cells. However each inversion was formed via a fairly precise reciprocal recombination event, with a minimal modification of sequences found at the breakpoint sites. These data favored direct induction of *RET*/PTC as a result of random double-strand DNA breaks, rather than disruption of the recombination machinery.

In addition, we observed that no long-sequence homology between regions of breakpoints in the *RET* and *ELE1* genes, indicating that this rearrangement is the result of illegitimate rather than homologous recombination (47).

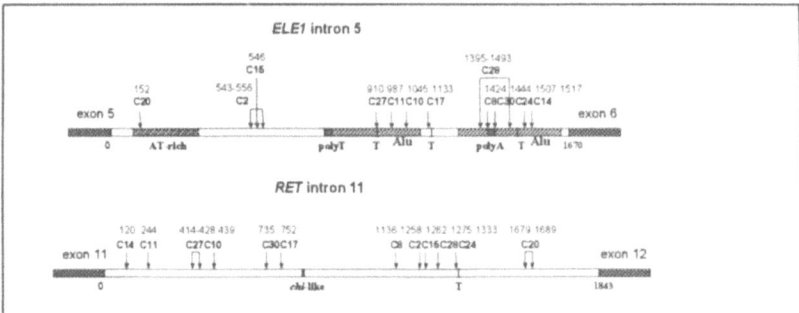

Fig. 3. *Distribution of breakpoints (arrows) in ELE1 and RET in 12 post-Chernobyl thyroid cancers with RET/PTC3 rearrangement. Poly-T and poly-A - polynucleotide sequences, Alu- Alu repeat, T- topo II recognition sequence. From (47).*

Thus, the breakpoints in the *ELE1* intron 5 and *RET* intron 11 were distributed in a relatively random fashion. However, upon further analysis of individual tumors, it was found that in each tumor the location of breakpoints in these two genes followed a certain pattern (47). After the alignment of the respective introns in opposite orientation, in each tumor the relative position of the breakpoint in one gene showed a correspondence to the location of the breakpoint on the other gene (Fig. 4). In 5/12 cases, the breakpoints were located just across from each other (Fig. 6,A). The other 7 pairs of breakpoints could be aligned by sliding one gene with respect to the other (Fig. 6,B,C). This predilection for breakpoint sites at one gene to correspond to a breakpoint site located within the certain region of the other gene suggests the presence of a stable spatial relationship between these two genomic regions within the nucleus. Thus, although the loci for *RET* and *ELE1* are at a considerable linear distance from each other (≥ 0.5 Mb), we hypothesized that in interphase nuclei they may be adjacent. This hypothesis also predict that generation of *RET*/PTC may be a direct effect of simultaneous DNA double-strand breaks produced by energy deposition of a single radiation track in two closely spaced DNA loci.

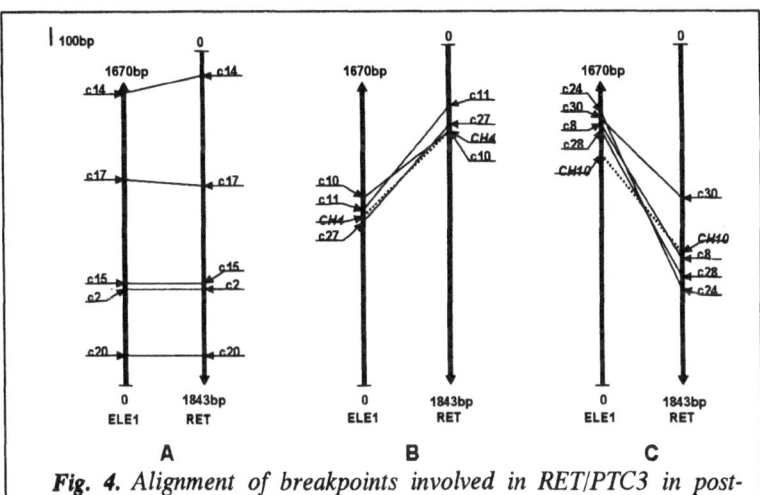

Fig. 4. Alignment of breakpoints involved in RET/PTC3 in post-Chernobyl tumors. From (47).

Since the *RET* and *ELE1* genes are on the same chromosome, the inter-action between these loci should involve chromosome folding. One of the levels of DNA packaging involves chromatin arrangement into loops of different size attached to a chromosomal backbone (Fig. 5) (49). Thus, although two chromosomal loci are located at a considerable linear distance from each other, they may be closely spaced in the interphase nucleus because of their location at specific areas of chromosomal loop(s) (forexample, points a and e or f and g, Fig. 5). Similarly, folding of chromosome 10 may result in approximation of the *ELE1* and *RET* genes (*RET*/PTC3) as well as *H4* and *RET* genes (*RET*/PTC1), that are located at 0.5 Mbp and 30 Mbp genomic separation respectively, in the nuclei of thyroid cells during certain stages of cell cycle.

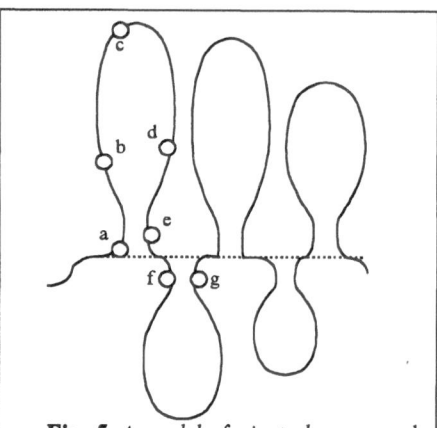

Fig. 5. *A model of giant chromosomal loops attached to a flexible backbone provided by the nuclear matrix/ scaffold (dotted line). From (49).*

Utilizing fluorescence in situ hybridization (FISH) with gene specific probes, we recently demonstrated the presence of spatial proximity between the *RET* and *H4* genes (50). We studied nuclear localization of *RET* and *H4* (*RET*/PTC1 partners) in primary cultured normal human thyroid follicular cells and compared it with nuclear localization of the *RET* and D10S539 probes. The latter locus was used as a control since it is located on chromosome 10q between *RET* and *H4* (51), and is not known to participate in a rearrangement. The analysis of 4 adult individuals revealed that in 35% of cells at least one pair of *RET* and *H4* loci were juxtaposed (Fig. 6) (50). By contrast, *RET* and D10S539 were juxtaposed in only 6% of nuclei.

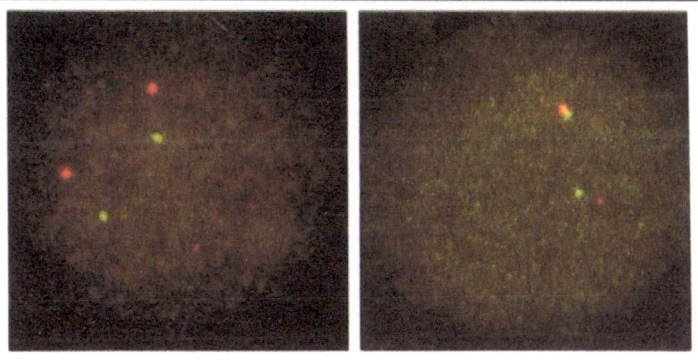

Fig. 6. *Interphase FISH with probes corresponding to the RET (green) and H4 (red) genes demonstrating two separately spaced pairs of genes (left), and one pair of juxtaposed signals (right) in the nuclei of normal thyroid follicular cells. Modified from (50).*

In addition, 2D interphase distances between *RET* - *H4* and *RET* - D10S539 were compared with a theoretical Rayleigh model that describes a distribution of 2D distances between two points of linear polymers that fold in a random manner. Previous studies have shown that interphase distances between random chromosomal loci that are greater than 10 Mb apart conform to the Rayleigh distribution (49,52). We found that *RET* - D10S539 distances conformed to the Rayleigh distribution, indicating random association between these two loci (Fig. 7). By contrast, RET and H4 distances showed dramatic deviation from the Rayleigh distribution (Fig. 7), primarily due to loci that were either juxtaposed or closer than expected, indicating that *RET* and *H4* are nonrandomly located with respect to each other. These data suggest that the preferential occurrence of *RET*/PTC rearrangements may be due in part to the structural organization of chromosome 10, resulting in the spatial proximity of potentially recombinogenic DNA sequences in the nuclei of normal human thyroid cells.

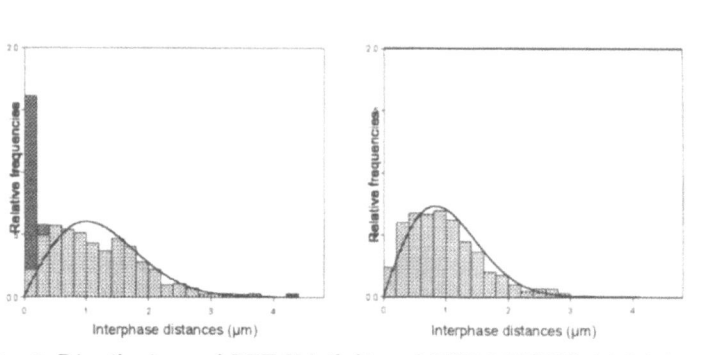

Fig. 7. *Distributions of RET-H4 (left) and RET-D10S539 (right) inter-phase distances as compared with the theoretical Rayleigh distribution (solid line). The distribution of RET-H4 distances strongly deviates form randomness with respect to distances 0 - <0.4 _m (black bars). Modified from (50).*

The juxtapositioning of *RET* and *H4* raised the question as to the whether interphase proximity of these loci is a general feature of human cells. This was studied in two additional cell types, peripheral blood lympho-cytes and mammary epithelial cells (50). Only lymphocytes showed *RET - H4* juxtaposition (21% of cells). This was confirmed by analysis of 2D interphase distances between *RET - H4* and *RET - D10S539* which showed that only *RET - H4* distances were not random in lymphocytes. Hence, the association between *RET* and *H4* is not a universal feature of human cells, although it is definitely present in cells other than the thy-roid.

If *RET - H4* proximity facilitates formation of *RET*/PTC1 in irradiated thyroid cells, then gene proximity would be implicated in susceptibility to radiation-induced cancer. The *RET*/PTC1 chimeric gene has been shown to be able to cause thyroid cancer and mammary cancer in trans-genic mice (53). Yet, *RET*/PTC1 rearrangements are not found in breast cancers in humans (54). In the light of our findings, it is reasonable to postulate that *RET*/PTC1 rearrangements in human mammary cells are rare because the *RET* gene is not usually near its translocation partner in these cells.

Our data also show that a high frequency of *RET - H4* juxtaposition can occur in human cells that are not known to suffer oncogenic *RET*/PTC1 rearrangements, i.e. lymphocytes. Data from transgenic mice expressing *RET*/PTC1 suggest an explanation. Although they have the

212

RET/PTC oncogene, these animals do not develop lymphomas, suggesting that lymphocytes may be resistant to *RET*/PTC-mediated transformation. Perhaps signaling through the *RET* tyrosine kinase is not sufficient for transformation of mouse lymphocytes. The same may be true in human lymphocytes.

These data suggest the following possible mechanism of *RET*/PTC generation after radiation exposure (Fig. 8). The *RET* gene and its translocation partner are located in close spatial proximity, but pointed in opposite directions in normal thyroid cells nuclei. The proximity may predispose them to be simultaneously damaged by a single radiation track so that free DNA ends have a high chance to be misrejoined at the same place in the nucleus, and this will lead to the rearrangement. This model would explain two findings: the high prevalence of *RET - H4* spatial proximity and the fact that the breakpoints in each tumor are often located just across from each other. Although we believe that this provides a structural basis for *RET*/PTC generation, much more should be learned to fully understand the role of gene proximity and chromosomal architecture in the generation of chromosomal rearrangements after radiation exposure.

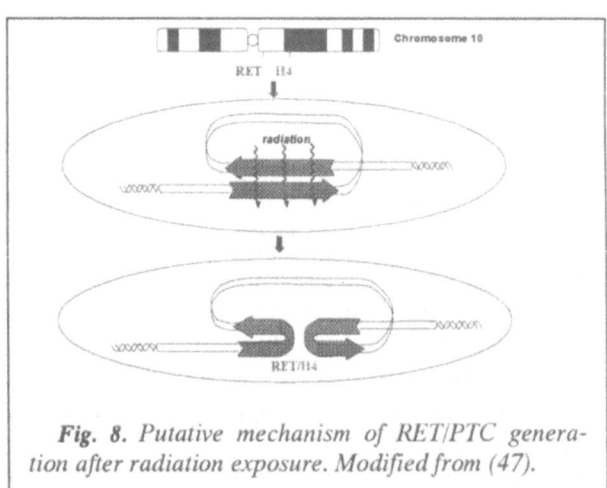

Fig. 8. *Putative mechanism of RET/PTC generation after radiation exposure. Modified from (47).*

Conclusions

1. *RET*/PTC rearrangements is the major genetic event in radiation-induced papillary thyroid carcinomas. Other mutations known in spo-

radic thyroid cancer, such as *RAS*, *p53*, and others, are rare in thyroid tumors associated with radiation exposure.

2. The *RET*/PTC3 type of rearrangement is more common in tumors arising after the short latent period (< 10 years); it is associated with the solid variant of papillary carcinoma.

3. *RET*/PTC3 rearrangements in these tumors result from illegitimate reciprocal recombination between the *RET* and *ELE1* genes.

4. Spatial proximity of the *RET*/PTC partners in interphase nuclei of normal thyroid follicular cells may provide a structural basis for generation of *RET* rearrangement via ligation of free DNA ends produced by radiation in two closely spaced chromosomal loci.

Acknowledgement

I would like to thank Marina Nikiforova and Amy Koshoffer who worked in my laboratory on spatial proximity of *RET*/PTC partner genes and on mapping of breakpoint sites, and James Fagin and James Stringer from the University of Cincinnati who were my invaluable collaborators on these projects.

References

1. Duffy, B.J., Jr. and Fitzgerald, P.J (1950) Cancer of the thyroid in children: a report of 28 cases. *J Clin Endocrinol Metab* 31: 1296-1308.

2. Winship, T. and Rosvoll, R.V (1970) Thyroid carcinoma in childhood: final report on a 20 year study. *Clinical Proceedings of Children's Hospital, Wasington, D.C.* 26: 327-348.

3. Mehta, M.P., Goetowski, P.G., and Kinsella, T.J (1989) Radiation induced thyroid neoplasms 1920 to 1987: a vanishing problem? *Int. J. Radiation Oncology Biol. Phys.* 16: 1471-1475.

4. Thompson, D.E., Mabuchi, K., Ron, E., et al (1994) Cancer incidence in atomic bomb survivors. Part II: Solid tumors, 1958-1987. *Radiation Research* 137: S17-S67.

5. Cronkite, E.P., Bond, V.P., and Conard, R.A (1995) Medical effects of exposure of human beings to fallout radiation from a thermonuclear explosion. *Stem cells* 13 (suppl 1):49-57.

6. Kerber, R.A., Till, J.E., Simon, S.L., et al (1993) A cohort study of thyroid disease in relation to fallout from nuclear weapons testing. *JAMA* 270: 2076-2082.

7. Gilbert, E.S., Tarone, R., Bouville, A., and Ron, E (1998) Thyroid cancer rates and ^{131}I doses from Nevada atmospheric nuclear bomb tests. *Journal of the National Cancer Institute* 90: 1654-1660.

8. Shneider, A.B., Ron, Ee., Lubin, J., Stovall, M., and Grierlowski, T.C. (1993) Dose-response relationships for radiation-induced thyroid cancer and thyroid nodules: Evidence for the prolonged effects of radiation on the thyroid. *J Clin Endocrinol Metab* 77: 362-369.

9. Shore, R.E., Hildreth, N., Dvoretsky, P., Andresen, E., Moseson, M., and Pasternack, B (1993) Thyroid cancer among persons given X-ray treatment in infancy for an enlarged thymus gland. *American Journal of Epidemiology* 137: 1068-10810.

10. Ron, E., Lubin, J.H., Shore, R.E., et al (1995) Thyroid cancer after exposure to external radiation: A pooled analysis of seven studies. *Radiation Research* 141: 259-277.

11. . Kazakov, V.S., Demidchik, E.P. and Astakhova, L.N (1992) Thyroid cancer after Chernobyl. *Nature* 359: 21.

12. Stsjazhko, V.A., Tsyb, A.F., Tronko, N.D., Souchkevitch, G., and Baverstock, K.F. (1995) Letter: Childhood thyroid cancer since accident at Chernobyl. *BMJ* 310: 80.

13. Pacini, F., Vorontsova, T., Demidchik,E.P., et al (1997) Post-Chernobyl thyroid carcinoma in Belarus children and adolescents: comparison with naturally occurring thyroid carcinoma in Italy and France. *J Clin Endocrinol Metab* 82: 3563-3569.

14. Nikiforov, Y. and Gnepp, D.R. (1994) Pediatric thyroid cancer after the Chernobyl disaster: Pathomorphologic study of 84 cases (1991-1992) from the Republic of Belarus. *Cancer* 74: 748-766.

15. Thomas GA, Bunnell H, Cook HA, et al (1999) High prevalence of *RET*/PTC rearrangements in Ukrainian and Belarussian post-Chernobyl thyroid papillary carcinomas: a strong correlation between *RET*/PTC3 and the solid-follicular variant. *J Clin Endocrinol Metab* 84:4232-38.

16. Nikiforov YE, Rowland JM, Bove KE, Monforte-Munoz H, Fagin JA. (1997) Distinct pattern of ret oncogene rearrangements in morphologic variants of radiation-induced and sporadic thyroid papillary carcinomas in children. *Cancer Res* 57: 1690-1694.

17. Fagin JA (1996) In: Werner and Ingbar's. *The Thyroid. A Fundamental and Clinical Text.* (Braverman, L.E., & Utiger, R.D., eds.), Lippincott-Raven, Philadelphia-New York 909-915.

18. Wright PA, Williams ED, Lemoine NR, Wynford-Thomas D (1991) Radiation-associated and 'spontaneous' human thyroid carcinomas

show a different pattern of ras oncogene mutation. *Oncogene* 16: 471-473.

19. Challeton C, Bounacer A, Du Villard JA, et al (1995) Pattern of ras and gsp oncogene mutations in radiation-induced human thyroid tumors. *Oncogene* 11: 601-603.

20. Nikiforov YE, Nikiforova M, Gnepp DR, Fagin JA (1996) Prevalence of mutations of *ras* and *p53* in thyroid tumors from children exposed to radiation after Chernobyl. *Oncogene* 13: 687-693.

21. Suchy B, Waldmann V, Klugbauer S, Rabes HM (1998) Absence of RAS and p53 mutations in thyroid carcinomas of children after Chernobyl in contrast to adult thyroid tumours. *Br J Cancer.* 77:952-955.

22. Santoro M, Thomas GA, Vecchio G, et al (2000) Gene rearrangement and Chernobyl related thyroid cancers. *Br J Cancer* 82, 315-322.

23. Fogelfeld LF, Bauer TK, Schneider AB, et al (1996) p53 mutations in radiation-induced thyroid cancer. *J Clin. Endocriol Metab* 81: 3039-3044.

24. Hillebrandt S, Streffer C, Reiners CHR, Demidchik E (1996) Mutations in the p53 tumour suppressor gene in thyroid tumours of children from areas contaminated by the Chernobyl accident. *Int. J.Radiat. Biol.* 69: 39-45.

25. Smida J, Zitzelsberger H, Kellerer AM, et al (1997) p53 mutations in childhood thyroid tumours from Belarus and in thyroid tumours without radiation history. *Int J Cancer* 73: 802-807.

26. Waldmann V, Rabes HM (1997) Absence of G(s)alpha gene mutations in childhood thyroid tumors after Chernobyl in contrast to sporadic adult thyroid neoplasia. *Cancer Res.* 57: 2358-2361.

27. Dubrova, Y.E., Nesterov, V.N., Krouchinsky, N.G., Ostapenko, V.A., (1996) Neumann, R., and Jeffreys, A.J. Human minisatellite mutation rate after the Chernobyl accident. *Nature* 380: 683-686.

28. Nikiforov, Y.E., Nikiforova, M. and Fagin, J.A (1998) Prevalence of minisatellite and microsatellite instability in radiation-induced post-Chernobyl pediatric thyroid carcinomas. *Oncogene* 17, 1983-1988.

29. Richter HE, Lohrer HD, Hieber L, Kellerer AM, Lengfelder E, Bauchinger M (1999) Microsatellite instability and loss of heterozygosity in radiation-associated thyroid carcinomas of Belarussian children and adults. *Carcinogenesis* 20: 2247-52.

30. Takahashi, M., Buma, Y., Iwamoto, T., Iaguma, Y., Ikeda, H., and Haiai, H (1988) Cloning and expression of the ret proto-oncogene

encoding a tyrosine kinase with two potential transmembrane domains. *Oncogene* 3: 571-578.

31. Grieco, M., Santoro, M., Berlingieri, M.T., et al (1990) PTC is a novel rearranged form of the ret proto-oncogene and is frequently detected in-vivo in human thyroid papillary carcinomas. *Cell* 60: 557-563.

32. Bongazone, I., Butti, M.G., Coronelli, S., et al (1994) Frequent activation of ret protooncogene by fusion with a new activating gene in papillary thyroid carcinomas. *Cancer Res* 54: 2979-2985.

33. Santoro, M., Dathan, N.A., Berlingieri, M.T (1994) Molecular characterization of RET/PTC3: a novel rearranged version of the RET proto-oncogene in a human thyroid papillary carcinoma. *Oncogene* 9: 509-516.

34. Bongarzone, I., Monzini, N., Borrello, M.G., et al (1993) Molecular characterization of a thyroid tumor-specific transforming sequence formed by the fusion of ret tyrosine kinase and the regulatory subunit RI_ of cyclic AMP-dependent Protein Kinase A. *Molecular and Cellular Biology* 13: 358-366.

35. Jhiang SM (2000) The RET proto-oncogene in human cancers. *Oncogene* 19: 5590-5597.

36. Klugbauer, S., Lengfelder, E., Demidchik, E.P., and Rabes, H.M (1995) High prevalence of RET rearrangement in thyroid tumors of children from Belarus after the Chernobyl reactor accident. *Oncogene* 11: 2459-2467.

37. Fugazzola, L., Pilotti, S., Pinchera, A., et al (1995) Oncogenic rearrangements of the RET proto-oncogene in papillary thyroid carcinomas from children exposed to the Chernobyl nuclear accident. *Cancer Res.* 55: 5617-5620.

38. Ito T, Seyama T, Iwamoto KS et al (1994) Activated RET oncogene in thyroid cancers of children from areas contaminated by Chernobyl accident. *Lancet* 344: 259.

39. Smida J, Salassidis K, Hieber L et al (1999) Distinct frequency of ret rearrangements in papillary thyroid carcinomas of children and adults from Belarus. *Int J Cancer* 80: 32-8.

40. Rabes HM, Demidchik EP, Sidorow JD et al (2000) Pattern of radiation-induced RET and NTRK1 rearrangements in 191 post-chernobyl papillary thyroid carcinomas: biological, phenotypic, and clinical implications. *Clin Cancer Res* 6: 1093-1103.

41. Bounacer, A., Wicker, R., Cailleux, A.F., Sarasin, A., Schlumgerger, M., and Suarez, H.G (1997) High prevalence of activating ret proto-

oncogene rearrangements, in thyroid tumors from patients who had received external radiation. *Oncogene* 15: 1263-1273.

42. Santoro M, Chiappetta G, Cerrato A, et al (1996) Development of thyroid papillary carcinomas secondary to tissue-specific expression of the RET/PTC1 oncogene in transgenic mice. *Oncogene* 12:1821-6.

43. Jhiang SM., Sagartz JE, Tong Q et al (1996) Targeted expression of the ret/PTC1 oncogene induces papillary thyroid carcinomas. *Endocrinology* 137: 375-378.

44. Powell, DJ Russell J, Niby K et al (1998) The RET/PTC3 oncogene: metastatic solid-type papillary carcinomas in murine thyroids. *Cancer Res.* 58: 5523-5528.

45. Ito, T., Seyama, T., Iwamoto, K.S., et al (1993) In vitro irradiation is able to cause RET oncogene rearrangement. Cancer Research, 53: 2940-2943

46. Mizuno, T., Kyoizumi, S., Suzuki, T., Iwamoto, K.S., and Seyama, T (1997) Continued expression of a tissue specific activated oncogene in the early steps of radiation-induced human thyroid carcinogenesis. *Oncogene* 15: 1455-1460.

47. Nikiforov, Y.E., koshoffer, A., Nikiforova, M., Stringer, J., and Fagin, J.A (1999) Chromosomal breakpoint positions suggest a direct role for radiation in inducing illegitimate recombination between the ELE1 and RET genes in radiation-induced thyroid carcinomas. *Oncogene* 18, 6330-6334.

48. Bongarzone, I., Butti, M.G., Fugazzola, L., et al (1997) Comparison of the breakpoint regions of ELE1 and RET genes involved in the generation fo RET/PTC3 oncogene in sporadic and in radiation-associated papillary thyroid carcinomas. *Genomics* 42: 252-259.

49. Yokota, H., van den Engh, G., Hearst, J.E., Sachs, R.K., and Trask, B.J (1995) Evidence for the organization of chromatin in megabase pair-sized loops arranged along a random walk path in the human GO/G1 interphase nucleus. *J Cell Biol* 130: 1239-1249.

50. Nikiforova MN, Stringer JR, Blough R, Medvedovic M, Fagin JA, and Nikiforov YE (2000) Proximity of chromosomal loci that participate in radiation-induced translocations in human cells. *Science* 290, 138-141.

51. Jossart, G.H., O'Brien, B., Cheng, J.-F., et al (1996) A novel multicolor hybridizaion scheme applied to localization of a transcribed sequence (D10S170/H4) and deletion mapping in the thyroid cancer cell line TPC-1. *Cytogenet. Cell Genet.* 75: 254-257.

52. Van den Engh, G, Sachs, R., and Trask, B.J (1992) Estimating genomic distance from DNA sequence location in cell nuclei by a random walk model. *Science* 257: 1410-1411.
53. Portella G, Salvatore D, Botti G, et al (1996) Development of mammary and cutaneous gland tumors in transgenic mice carrying the RET/PTC1 oncogene. *Oncogene* 13: 2021-6.
54. Santoro M, Sabino N, Ishizaka Y, et al (1993) Involvement of RET oncogene in human tumours: specificity of RET activation to thyroid tumours. *Br J Cancer* 68: 460-4.

Key Word Index